Cancer Widow, Cancer Survivor

Rita K Miller Kasinskas

Rita K Miller Kasinskas
6/14/2024

A Roar A Publishing

A-ROAR-A
PUBLISHING

Cover design by: Rachel Kasinskas Tourville
Library of Congress Control Number: 2018675309
Printed in the United States of America

This book is dedicated to the memory of my husband Tom Kasinskas who not only shared my life but our journey through cancer.

I also wish to dedicate this book to my children, Phillip, Rachel, and Valerie, who also took this journey with us.

To my sisters, Lindalee, Sandy, and Valerie Jean and my dear friend, Kathy, who's presence helped us to make this journey with great support and dignity.

"In Cancer Widow, Cancer Survivor, author Rita Kasinskas opens up a personal journal describing her initial battle and recovery from cancer as well as her husband's subsequent diagnosis, treatments and death from cancer. Her struggle will be familiar to both cancer patients and those that care for patients with cancer. As she describes her journey, she weaves in valuable information regarding cancer, it's diagnosis and treatment: information that would be helpful to any patient newly diagnosed with cancer. Health care professionals will gain a powerful understanding of how a diagnosis of cancer affects a family. Cancer survivors will particularly find helpful the action plans she found useful as she moved on with life after her husband's death."
Randy Hurley M. D. Oncology

"Cancer Widow, Cancer Survivor details the emotional journey of a cancer victim suddenly changing roles to cancer caregiver of her husband, and unfortunately becoming a widow. This book presents a truly honest account of the struggles of changing family dynamics and navigation of the unknown medical world, along with helpful tips for others facing cancer. Throughout the pages, it continues to amaze me the inner strength people discover on their road to becoming a cancer survivor."
Linda Austin RN OCN

CONTENTS

INTRODUCTION
CONTENT OF CHAPTERS

FORWARD

By Lindalee A. Miller-Nelson

How we approach our challenges in life show in our personal journey as we walk upon this earth. Each person has a story to tell. Each person uses the tools and experiences that they collect over their lives to move forward and through the next journey.

Rita has taken all her experiences, challenges, wisdom, endurance, and perseverance and wrote this book on a huge chapter in her life that changed every fiber of her being. From a life full of husband, children, family, career and friends into titles such as cancer survivor, widow, disabled, single parent, caregiver, sole provider, and facing a future that had to be rewritten.

First being diagnosed with cancer herself and then having her husband, Tom, diagnosed with cancer soon after, took a monumental amount of courage to keep moving forward with stamina, faith, and the workings of all her past experiences to face everything that was being thrown at her at once.

Rita's ability to express all she lived through and continues to live through, is present in her ability to do extensive research about the cancers, and to dig deep to accomplished sound conclusions in all areas of her life, and to trust and surround herself and her loved ones with family, caregivers and excellent medical staff to fight the battle.

This book will take you through her journey filled with the depth of her being to share with you what took place, day by day, and how she pushed forward keeping her faith and her drive to fight each day for herself and her family. It covers how she approaches the first emotional moment of her diagnosis: "You have cancer" and then, "Tom has terminal cancer". On to the long journey of treatments, hospitals, and doctors, losses and wins.

Her ability to describe in detail this journey will help anyone who picks up this book and a dose of courage.

Rita shares the fiber of their personal lives and how it affected their complete world with hope and compassion.

As Rita writes: " I learned that life is not always easy, but life is worth living."

Lindalee A. Miller-Nelson is the author of
"Patrick and The Little Red Wagon"

PREFACE

Cancer Widow, Cancer Survivor reflects a journey as a couple, for Tom and I after we both received a diagnosis of cancer only five months apart. The journey is presented through a daily journal format, sharing the events of our lives as they unfolded. The challenges, heartaches, success, and setbacks are presented in a first-person style, bringing the reader wholly into our lives.

I learned to accept help from others during radiation and chemotherapy treatments, while my husband, Tom showed his love and support by becoming my caregiver.

Only five months later, Tom receives a diagnosis of terminal cancer as I accepted the added role as a caregiver for Tom during my recovery.

Definitions of treatments, tests, nutritional needs, and personal insights are presented within the dialogue, giving the reader helpful answers as each process occurs.   This knowledge and understanding gives the reader valuable information in their search for answers.

After Tom loses his fifteen-month battle with cancer, I continue sharing my life as I struggled to recover as a widow and cancer survivor while adjusting to physical limitations resulting from cancer and treatments.

My journey continues as I share my process, the guilt of my cancer survivorship, being a widow, and the ways I discovered to adjust to my new physical limitations. I share personal insights and helpful techniques that gave me strength to endure and the skills to learn to live without Tom.

May my inspirations offer hope and encouragement to cancer survivors, caregivers, widow or widowers and people with newly acquired physical limitations.

Even though the book concludes, I have indeed discovered that I can live a full and complete life in the wake of my extreme changes, I realize that life is valuable and worth the struggle to survive.

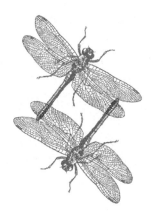

CHAPTER 1 - IN SICKNESS AND IN HEALTH

When people are faced with extreme challenges, we cannot avoid wondering why me? I personally feel there is no true answer to that question, no matter how many times I asked. One of my greatest challenges in life was surviving cancer. There is more to surviving cancer than defeating the disease; it is also surviving what comes after treatments. For me, the challenge was not only my cancer, but my husband's cancer as well.

In September of 2004 when I was diagnosed with cancer, I was faced with the challenge of this question, why me? Five months later, when my husband also received a diagnosis of cancer, this question haunted me greater than it had with my diagnoses.

Yet, I still have not found the answer to this question, but I have learned that there was strength, endurance, and survival within me that I did not know I had. I experienced cancer from both sides. I went from being a cancer patient to a cancer patient and caregiver, as my husband went from being a cancer caregiver to being a cancer patient.

The love Tom and I had shared for over twenty-seven years laid the foundation for each of us, as we faced the challenges of our own cancers, and both of us as we dealt with both our cancers as a couple. Love is the most powerful weapon against cancer, providing strength, endurance, and stamina, as we fought this devastating intruder into our lives.

Tom and I met while he was attending college at UW Stout. I was living in St. Paul, but both of our parents lived in Gordon, Wisconsin. We both happen to be visiting our parents the weekend we met. The notion of love at first sight became a reality to me the day we met. He seemed to be a person I wanted to get to know better

A week after we met, I received a letter from Tom expressing how much he enjoyed meeting me and inviting me to stop by the summer dorms at Stout anytime I was in the neighborhood. Anxious to see him again, I drove to the dorms to look him up. After I arrived, he asked what I was doing in Menomonie. I immediately felt that I may have been being to forward by looking him up. I quickly made up an excuse that I was on my way to Eau Claire to register for vocational school. Being kindhearted, he offered to go with me and help me with my registration. What could I do? That day I became a registered student at the vocational school in Eau Claire.

Becoming a student became very beneficial to our relationship. We began to see each other on weekends and spent time together in Gordon. Our love for each other began to grow with each passing week. By the January semester, I was accepted as a student of psychology at UW Stout. Tom and I rented a trailer house together. Soon our lives became more entwined as time journeyed on.

Upon our engagement, Tom told me he did not want to get married until he was out of college for one year. He graduated May 18, 1978, and our wedding date was May 19, 1979. He got his year.

I was nervous on our wedding day. We were making a lifelong commitment to each other to share all that life would bring our way. My hands were sweaty and trembling as I tried to steady my shaking ring finger as Tom lovingly placed the wedding band on it. As the simple gold band took its perman-ent place upon my finger, I recalled those two little words "I do" which changed my life forever; representing the bond of our en-during love for each other and the beginning of a future of hopes and dreams, that Tom and I would share for a lifetime.

The power of simple words or phrases, which can quickly change your life, amazes me. When my husband and I married, we spoke those simple words, "I do" that bound us together for life. Within our vows, there were yet other simple words that would bind us together even further.

Those simple words, heard at most weddings, "For better or for worse, in sickness and in health." Little did I know, on one the most joyous day of our lives, to what depth those words would test our love and our marriage.

Our wedding day was one of the most memorable and enjoyable days of our lives. Whenever I think of that day, I say, "It's the best party I have ever attended". Nature had complied by giving us a beautiful Wisconsin spring day. It was more then we could have ever hoped. Everything was perfect.

Adventures waited us as we eventually moved to Ken-tucky, which provided Tom with a new employment op-portunity. Kentucky was breathtaking lined with white fences engulfing safe havens for the magnificent horses, the pride of Kentucky. Even though our stay in Kentucky was relatively short, we received a great blessing in November of 1980. Our son Phillip, whose name means "lover of horses", was born.

I must admit that even though our wedding was truly joyous, it paled compared to the day Phillip was born. I did not realize that the heart could experience such an abundance of joy all at once.

Early the next spring an opening within the company Tom worked for, transported us back to Wisconsin. I must admit I was homesick. I missed family, friends, and the wonder-ful variety of the four seasons that the Midwest bestowed.

Tom loved the water. He enjoyed fishing, water skiing and canoeing. We were fortunate enough to find property on the north end of a small but serene lake. While we were building our new house, I discovered that I was pregnant. Unplanned events sometimes become the most powerful and memorable. We had planned to wait until the house was done, but nature decided a different timeline for us.

On September 3, 1982, one month early, our lovely daughter Rachel was born. Eight minutes later, quite unexpectedly, our equally lovely daughter, Valerie was born. We had no idea we were having twins. Some surprises come in cute little packages.

We had our share of "For better or for worse" and some "In sickness and in health". Treasures, such as our children, become more valued when the threat of losing them arises. At ten weeks of age, while driving for a Thanksgiving visit to Gordon, Rachel stopped breathing. Tom quickly pulled the car over and took Rachel from me. The hot tears streamed down my face as Tom attempted to get Rachel to breathe. After she started breathing again, Tom took us immediately to a local hospital. She was red faced and screaming because she had missed her feeding and was demanding her meal.

The ER doctor said he suspected Infant Sleep Apnea. We made a detour to the girls' pediatrician in Menomonie and discussed the possibility of this condition. Infant sleep Apnea is more common in premature babies usually due to the physical immaturity of their premature birth. The girls were placed on Infant Apnea monitors and after quick instructions on their use, we ventured back to Gordon.

The girl's baptism was to take place at the same church where Tom and I were married, and where Phillip had been baptized. The apnea monitors went off frequently, signaling that one of them had stopped breathing and I was panicky. After calling the girls' doctor, he suggested that we go to St. Paul for a more in-depth follow-up care. In the middle of our well-laid plans, we found ourselves witnessing our daughters' baptism in the middle of my parent's living room before journeying one hundred and thirty-five miles in an ice storm to a children's hospital in St. Paul.

After test and days in the hospital, both of our daughters were diagnosed with Infant Sleep Apnea. We finally went home with high quality training relating to Infant Sleep Apnea, state of the art monitors and reassurance that our precious daughters would survive. Ten months later, the girl's systems became mature enough for them to shed the monitors and begin a normal life.

In the meantime, Phillip developed asthma and allergies. We handled this situation and learned about yet another condition of childhood. Tom and I leaned on each other, and our love nurtured each of us so we could endure whatever our lives together offered.

Illnesses, broken bones, school awards, dating and finally graduations carried us along on our journey of life. Love kept us forever strong.

Rachel and Valerie moved onto college, UW Stout, majoring in Art. Phillip remained living with us as he contemplated attending some type of college. All in all, the independence of our children gave Tom and me more time for each other.

Tom and I filled up the empty nest hours restoring classic cars. It had been one of Tom's hobbies before we had met. I have always enjoyed a good muscle car and my dad taught me to be a fair mechanic. I was as excited as Tom.

The first car we restored was a 1971 Boss 351 Mustang fastback. It took almost two years to restore the Mustang, during which Tom and I shared the best quality time we could have hoped. In May 2002, we took the car to our first car show. The next two summers provided many car shows and many trophies. It was great fun. Our life together was fulfilling the hopes and dreams that began the day we were married. Unfortunately, things can change at the spur of the moment. The true test of our marriage vows came rudely and abruptly in September of 2004.

Flexible Sigmoidoscopy

August 2004

As we deal with everyday aches and pains, occasionally things out of the normal do arise. Sometimes we ignore them or sometimes we receive the wrong medical advice. The two years prior to my cancer diagnosis, my bowel problems were haunting, often resulting in severe constipation. I felt bloated with bowel movements streaked with blood. I had undergone two Flexible Sigmoidoscopy exams over the years. This is a visual exam of rectum and sigmoid colon. The sigmoid colon is just above the rectum. A lighted, flexible tube with an eyepiece is used to look at this area.

My first exam in 1989 was insignificant meaning nothing to worry about existed. The one in April 1997 indicated a lesion on the lower left quadrant of my anal area. My doctor calmly said, "It's insignificant and nothing, don't worry about it." Therefore, I did not and neither did she. Little did I know how crucial her use of "insignificant" was to become. She simply recommended that I add more roughage to my diet.

No matter how much roughage I added, the constipation, pain and bleeding problem continued to worsen. The problem continued while my doctor continued to give me the same advice. Nothing improved.

By March 2004, often, the toilet filled with blood when I had a bowel movement. I continued to express my concerns with my doctor. Without even an exam, she suggested that I had a bleeding hemorrhoid. Again, she suggested I continue to add more roughage to my diet. The constipation and bleeding continued. I was becoming worried.

Finally, in August of 2004, I did a self-exam. I was shocked at what I felt. I was convinced that it was not a hemorrhoid. Hemorrhoids are swollen blood vessels, and this did not feel that way to me. It was more solid than I thought a hemorrhoid would feel. I spoke to my husband about it.

"Tom, I did a self-exam of that sore in my rectum, and I am very concerned about it."

"What do you mean, concerned?" he asked.

"The doctor said it was a bleeding hemorrhoid. I thought a hemorrhoid was soft and squishy, but this isn't."

Tom laughed at my use of words.

"I don't know," he replied, "Just go to the doctor and get it checked out. Then you won't have to keep worrying about it."

I made an appointment to see my doctor.

When my doctor entered the exam room, she was seemingly supportive. I had been seeing her for over twenty years.

"What seems to be the problem today?" she asked.

"I am concerned about the hemorrhoid I have. I did a self-exam and I do not think it is a hemorrhoid. I want you to look at it and tell me what it is."

I slipped into exam gown and rolled over onto my side.

Upon examination, she commented that she agreed with me and that the problem area did not seem to be a hemorrhoid at all. She decided that I needed a colonoscopy and a biopsy of that area.

I had taken my father for his colonoscopy and understood the procedure. My appointment was set up for August 18, 2004. That week I received directions and information about the test and preparation instructions.   I was surprised at how quickly I had gotten an appointment. It was only two weeks away.

After I confirmed the appointment, I remembered that my sister, Sandy, from Oregon was going to be here for a visit since one of our nieces was getting married. I was going to be Sandy's sole means of getting around while she was visiting.

I called her to talk about my recent doctor appointment.

"Hi Sandy, this is Rita. The doctor doesn't think it's a hemorrhoid and wants me to have a colonoscopy."

"That's a good idea, and then you can find out what it is and not have to worry about it anymore", she said.

"I know. The problem is that my test is while you are here. I think I should change it to a later date."

She sighed. "You know how long it takes to get tests set up. You were lucky to get it so soon. I would not change it. We

can work around it."
I kept the appointment.

Colonoscopy
Wednesday, August 18, 2004

A colonoscopy is an examination of the large intestine or colon, which can be four to six feet in length and includes portions of the small bowel. An instrument called an endoscope is used for this exam.   It is a long, thin flexible instrument connected to a camera and provides internal viewing with the use of a video display monitor.

Once the instrument is inserted into the rectum, it is gently moved through the colon. Sometimes abnormal growths, called polyps, are found, and removed. This instrument is also used to remove polyps or to take a biopsy of suspicious tissues.

Polyps are growth of abnormal tissues protruding from the colon mucus membranes. Not all polyps are cancerous and are removed to reduce the likelihood of becoming cancer.

The preparation for a colonoscopy has one major goal. The goal is to clean the entire length of the large colon. There are several prep kits used for this purpose and the doctor conducting the exam will decide on the prep you will use.

Preparation for the test was one of the worse experiences I have ever had. The texture and awful flavor of the prep was a traumatic struggle for me.

The prep is an oral laxative solution, diluted in a glass of liquid such as water or broth. Then at timed intervals, you drink the entire glass of liquid laxative. Drinking the solution is not such an easy task as I felt the flavor was the most awful thing I had ever put past my lips. The prep I had, required six glasses or a total of one gallon of solution. The over-powering taste of salt was unbearable to me. I tried mixing it with flavored drinks, the next one juice and still another one with chicken broth. I will never drink chicken broth again!

Drinking a gallon of the fowl-tasting laxative was a chore. By the time I got to the fifth glass, I was crying during my efforts to swallow it. Finally, I just added a small amount of water to the remaining solution and chugged it. I chased it with a full glass of water. That went much better. I was overjoyed when I had finally finished.

Of course, the solution did its job quite well. By morning, my colon was squeaky clean, and I was ready for the exam.

Even though the preparation for this exam is uncomfortable to undertake, the importance and possible life saving benefits of the exam is well worth a few hours of discomfort.

Since the drug given during the exam caused drowsiness, my son Phillip took me. I did not find the exam overly uncomfortable. The relaxation medication helped quite a bit.

The doctor talked to me as she conducted the test. She informed me that my colon and bowel looked very good. She expressed that it was on of the healthiest ones she had seen. She did however express her concern for the area just inside my anus. She took several biopsies of this area to send to the lab and told me she would put a three-day rush on it.

I was a little groggy when my son came from the waiting room to sit with me while I recovered.

"How are you doing, mom?"

"I'm pretty good. I am glad it's over."

After being in recovery for about an hour, we went home and began the wait for the tests results.

Waiting for the test results was the hardest. Whenever I mentioned my concern to anyone, they all had the same answer.

"I wouldn't worry about it, it's probably nothing."

I really found that statement overused. Why does it have to be nothing? People are diagnoses with cancer all the time. So far, I felt that our family had been quite fortunate. In a family circle of over sixty people, only two received a diagnosis of cancer.

One was my mother's mother or my grandmother. The other was my father's uncle John. Both died from their cancer, but in both cases, the cancer had progressed greatly before it was discovered. This emphasizes the important of early detection, which greatly increases survival rates.

I thought I was prepared for the answer, no matter, which one, yes or no. I felt strong and healthy and believed I would be able to handle what may come. Besides, if one of our family members had to have cancer, I would rather it was I.

Test Results
Wednesday, September 1, 2004

The three-day rush on my biopsies turned into a two and a half week wait. I called the doctor who did my exam several times over the past two weeks with no reply. One day, when the phone rang, I did not expect it to be the doctor who conducted the test. Her voice was detached as she said, "I have your test results. I am sorry to tell you that it is positive for cancer."

I was utterly shocked when I heard the words and realized that I was not as prepared to hear them as I had thought. As tears began to fall down my cheeks, my chest felt tight, making it difficult to breathe, I asked, "What do I do now?"

Her reply was blunt and to the point.

"You can have radiation and chemotherapy, have surgery or you can do nothing and die."

Her last words threw me for a loop and seemed like a strange thing to say.

"Who do I talk to now? Does my regular doctor have the results yet?"

"She has a copy of the report. Call her and talk to her about what you want to do next."

I hung up the phone and I started to cry. A sudden wave of fear surged throughout my body. Cancer! I have cancer. I thought to myself, "I always thought I would live forever or at least until I was one hundred. Now what do I have two or three years?"

I cried and cried as I thought about calling Tom at work. I finally pulled myself together, wiped my tears and dialed the phone.

No matter how hard I tried, I could not keep from crying

as I told him the news.

"The doctor called." I could hardly get the words out of my mouth. "I have cancer," and started to sob.

Tom's voice was calm. "I'll call you back in a few minutes."

Those few minutes seemed like hours. Finally, the phone rang, and it was Tom.

"I am on my way home. I love you."

It was very difficult to wait for Tom to get home. What were we going to say to each other? How do you make someone feel better after this type of news?

I stared at the ceiling with tears cascading everywhere as I waited for Tom to get home. I did not want to think, and I did not want to feel.

Tom entered the house quickly embracing me within his arms. As he hugged me, he allowed himself to cry. There we stood in our living room, holding each other, and crying.

After we comforted each other for a while, I could tell that Tom was full of questions.

"What type of cancer is it?"

"I don't know."

"What are we supposed to do next?"

I repeated what the doctor had said.

Tom was upset.

"What kind of an answer is that? Have you called your doctor yet?'

"No not yet. I'll do that now", I said.

Tom sat patiently as I called the clinic.

I told the nurse I wanted to talk to my personal doctor and wondered if she were in. I told her that I just found out I have cancer and I don't know what to do next."

The nurse took my name and number.

"I will have her call you as soon as she can."

I sheepishly smiled at Tom.

"She'll call me back. What do we do now?"

We both sat quietly for a while, neither of us knowing what to say. What do we say? It is going to be OK. Do we say?

Do not worry; it will all be taken care of. It seemed the unknown was worse than the known. We knew I had cancer, but no idea of what cell type. Even if we did know the cell type, it did not mean anything to us, since we knew absolutely nothing about cancer, except people die from it.

About ten minutes later the phone rang.

"Hello."

"Hello, Rita." It was my personal doctor. "How are you doing?"

"I'm not sure. I just found out I have cancer."

"Yes. I know. I'm sorry." She paused. "Did you say you just found out today? I've had the test results for over a week."

I felt betrayed by her for not telling me the tests results herself and especially since, she had the results for over a week.

"I was supposed to get the results over a week ago, but the colonoscopy doctor just called me today. I'd been calling her all week."

"I was wondering why you hadn't called me to discuss treatments."

"Because no one called to let me know I had cancer." I replied. Then I asked, "What type of cancer is it?"

"You have invasive squamous cell carcinoma."

"What do we do now?" I asked.

She replied, "We have an oncologist who comes to Baldwin once a month. His name is Dr. H., and he will be here tomorrow. I will make an appointment for you. One of his nurses will call you today with the time. I just want to say again how sorry I am to hear about your cancer."

"I'm sorry too. I'll wait for the call about the appointment."

Telling Family

As I hung up the phone, I realized that we needed to tell our children about the cancer diagnosis. I rubbed my face with my shaking hands. I suddenly filled with terror. I needed to tell our children.

"How do we tell the kids that I have cancer? This is crummy timing. Two days from now is Rachel and Valerie's birthday."

Tom put his arms around me and silently held me close for a few minutes. His release was just as gentle.

"Give them a call and ask them to come home because you have something to tell them."

Telling your loved ones that you have cancer is a very difficult thing to do. How do you prepare them for the news? I had absolutely no idea. I was not sure if this type of thing should be told to someone over the phone. I felt cheated when the doctor told me over the phone. It would have seemed more appropriate if she had told me in person. However, she was not my regular doctor and did not even know me. She probably told people daily that they had cancer.

A few minutes later, the phone rang. It was the clinic. My appointment with Dr. H. was at 8:20 a.m. the next morning. I felt a sense of relief knowing that we were already starting the process of doing something to treat my cancer. I know Tom could see the worry on my face.

Tom sat next to me holding my hand.

"We'll beat this thing. I want to grow old with you," Tom said.

Those loving words embedded themselves within my heart. I repeated them many times throughout my treatments as a source of strength. "I want to grow old with you."

Our son was still living with us, so when he came home, I swallowed hard and greeted him at the door.

"Hi, Phillip, how was work?"

"It was work," he replied.

"Can you sit down for a minute? I have something to tell you."

He sat on the couch and sighed. He did not even give me a chance to get the words out.

"You have cancer, don't you?" he said.

I started to cry.

"Yes," I replied.

He got up from the couch and hugged me.

"Don't worry mom, you'll beat it."

"I know I will, but I am still afraid."

"If you need me to take time off work to drive you to the doctor, just let me know. I still have some personal time I can take," Phillip said.

"Thank you. I probably will."

He gave me a gentle hug. "Now you have to tell the girls."

"The girls" were our twin daughters, Rachel, and Valerie, who were attending the UW-Stout, only thirty-five miles away. It was an easy drive home.

I looked pleadingly first to Phillip and them Tom. "Should I tell them over the phone?"

Phillip spoke first.

"Tell them you want them to come home so you can talk to them."

Tom handed me the phone.

I dialed their number, still uncertain if I was going to tell them on the phone or not. If I asked them to come home two days earlier than we had planned, they would suspect it anyway. I was leaning toward telling them right away.

Rachel answered the phone.

"Hi, Rachel, this is mom."

"Oh! Mom! Hi! How are you?"

"I'm OK. I have something I need discuss with you and Valerie. Can you come home for a visit?" I paused for a moment. Before I could continue, Rachel interrupted.

"You got your test results back, didn't you?"

"Yes, I did."

"Do you have cancer?" she asked.

"Yes, I do."

There was silence on the other end of the line.

Then Rachel spoke.

"It will be OK. Mom, I love you. We'll get a nutrition program and some good herbs, and you'll beat it."

"I know I will. I love you too. Is Val there?"

"She's at work. Do you want me to tell her?"

"Do you want to?"

"Yes." Rachel replied. "We will come over tomorrow. I will look up whatever I can on natural cancer cures, and we will get a good program for you. I love you."

"I love you too. I must call Sandy and grandma and let them know. I will talk to you later. Love you."

"Love you too. Bye."

As I hung up the phone, I was both relieved I had told her, but apprehensive about the cancer. Rachel and Valerie are big into nutrition and organic eating. I knew they would come up with a good nutrition program geared toward fighting cancer.

My sister Sandy in Oregon was the next person I called.

After sharing the news with her, she responded, "Aren't you glad you didn't cancel your appointment? It could have gotten so much worse."

I knew she was right.

"Sandy, could you call Lindalee and Val for me so I can call mom and dad? It is so hard to keep saying. Would you do that for me?"

"Yes, I will. Love you" Sandy replied.

"Love you too."

Lindalee is my oldest sister and Val is my youngest sister. Val is the namesake for my daughter Valerie.

Telling my parents about my cancer was a blur. I dreaded it because my mom still had not gotten over the loss of her mother from cancer. I hated telling her. Their voices seemed calm as I told them the news. My mom assured me that I was strong and could beat it. I told her I would.

Tom took on the task of telling his family. It is exceedingly difficult to repeat everything over, and over again. It sinks in deeper and deeper each time you repeat it or hear it. By the time I had told my family, and Tom had told his, I was sick of hearing it, sick of repeating it. I wanted it all to "just go away".

With Rachel and Valerie's birthday in just two days and I

felt guilty that this type of news would overshadow the joy of their twenty-second birthday.

I called my best friend, Kathy and told her of my diagnosis. She was supportive and offered to help in any way she could. She had a good idea of what I was going through since her sister had survived colon cancer just one year earlier.

After the phone calls, I was emotionally exhausted. I did not want to think or talk cancer anymore.

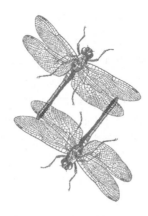

CHAPTER 2 - RITA'S DIAGNOSIS

Thursday, September 2, 2004

Tom and I arrived a little early for my appointment with the Oncologist. While we sat in the waiting room, horrible thoughts of chemotherapy filled my mind. The only thing I knew about cancer was from tales of "old" and a movie I had seen about a man's struggle with chemotherapy. He was sick most of the time and seemed as though misery was an everyday thing in his life.

I was not looking forward to that. I seemed to be jumping the gun. My appointment with the Oncologist would answer many of my questions.

Oncologist

An oncologist is a doctor who specializes in the study and treatment of cancerous tumors. Your Oncologist becomes your primary health care provider. All treatments such as chemotherapy and radiation are coordinated through your Oncologist. Side effects such as pain, nausea, and fatigue you will also discuss with your Oncologist. Some have areas of specialties such as a gynecological oncologist or a surgical oncologist.

Tom and I sat quietly for the doctor to come in.

The first few moments after the doctor came into the room, he seemed threatening to me, but I realized it was not the doctor I felt threatened by, it was the cancer.

My impression soon became a good one, which made me feel more comfortable about having a new doctor. His voice was gentle as was his mannerism. I imagined that he dealt with people with cancer daily and had an in depth understanding of patients' nervousness and fears.

He sat on a chair near Tom and me and began to explain my cancer to us.

"You have invasive Squamous cell carcinoma, which is a form of skin cancer," he explained.

My facial expression let him know that I was surprised that skin cancer could grow inside. He explained that skin cancer can form on any skin area, including the ones inside, such as inside your nose, throat, lungs, and your anus.

He then asked me how my cancer was discovered. I explained to him my most recent health history, which lead up to the colonoscopy and my present health status. I explained to him the results of my most recent flexi exam that revealed the lesion at the site of my present cancer. I also stated that my personal doctor did not address it. She simply said it was nothing and not to worry about it.

We continued by discussing my present prescriptions and any vitamins or supplements I was taking. Dr. H. did not see any necessary changes with my vitamin program. It is important for the doctor to know what you are taking because some supplements interfere with cancer treatments.

He further explained that he was going to treat my cancer with both radiation and chemotherapy. He said it would be a very aggressive treatment but felt that it is the best plan.

"How old are you?" he asked.

"I'm fifty years old." I replied.

"The reason I'm asking is that we don't even start screening for this type of cancer until people are well over fifty. Do you have any siblings?"

"Yes, three sisters."

"Since this could run in the family, all of your sisters should have a colonoscopy as soon as possible."

Dr. H. returned to the subject of treatment.

"I am going to set you up for an appointment for an anal ultra-sound to determine the size and stage of your cancer."

An Anal Ultrasound is an exam using a probe to view inside the anal area.

He continued, "I will also set you up with an appointment with a radiologist in St Paul. He is very good."

He further explained that he wished he could tell me more about my chances of a cure.

"It's one of the first thing patients want to know. Right now, I would like to tell you that your chances are good. About eight five percent, but I will know more after your ultra-sound. Right now, I want to do a chest x-ray to make sure the cancer has not metastasized to your lungs."

He explained that metastasis meant that the cancer from a primary cancer moves to other parts of the body.

I found that information disturbing. I had not even considered that this might have happened.

While I left to go to radiology, his nurse, Linda, began setting up appointments for me. My head was swirling from information over-load as I walked to the radiation department. Once the chest x-ray was complete, I returned to the exam room where my husband sat quietly.

What seemed like a lifetime later, Dr. H. returned to the room with his nurse.

"Good news, no sign of any cancer in your lungs. We will do a CT scan next Tuesday to make sure it hasn't metastasized to any other part of your body."

Since Dr. H. came to our local clinic only once or twice a month, my next appointment with him would be in St. Paul at the cancer center located in his primary hospital. He assured us that he would have all the test results and we could begin treatment right away.

He squeezed my hand and smiled.

"I'll see you then." He left the room and his nurse, Linda, sat down to talk with us.

My appointment with the radiation oncologist was set up for Wednesday, September 8, at the radiation therapy center was at the same hospital for one o'clock p.m. My appointment was with Dr. B.

While my nurse, Linda had been talking on the phone with the Pelvic Floor Disorders clinic, they were interested in having me participate in a clinical study during my exam.

I looked at her wondering what she meant.

"A seminar for pelvic floor disorders is going on next week and they are interested in having patients be a part of it," she explained. "They said they would do the test for free if you participate."

She explained that the ultrasound would be filmed and simultaneously viewed on a closed-circuit camera and be viewed by over 250 doctors. My participation would serve to educate doctors about cancer of the anus and offer firsthand information.

Tom and I looked at each other as though we had the same thought. We agreed it was a good idea for research and it would save us some money.

"Sure. I'll do it."

She returned a call to the disorders clinic and set the time and date I would participate.

My anal ultrasound exam was set up at ten o'clock Wednesday, September 8, during the seminar at a local Minneapolis hotel convention center. They promised to have the test results to Dr. B before my appointment with him in the afternoon.

I sighed as I mustered a smile. "OK, I guess we are all set."

After we left the clinic, I barely remember the ride home. I really did not want to talk about any of it. I knew it would not go away if I did not talk, but it helped me not to think about it so much.

Nutrition and Supplements

Later that night Rachel and Valerie came for a visit a day early. They were armed with vitamins, minerals, and a nutritional program for me. They are so loving and kind, and it warmed my heart. Just their presence gave me strength.

"How are you, mom?" They both asked at the same time. Our twin daughters often did this. We called it their "stereo response" one from each speaker!

"Mom," Rachel began. "We've done a lot of research and have found some information we want to share with you. There are a lot of natural things you can do to help you get through this."

Valerie continued the conversation.

"We think you should try a natural cure instead of radiation and chemotherapy."

I was touched by their passion and belief in natural cures for many things, but my uncertainties or lack of faith kept me from being enthusiastic about approaching cancer based solely on natural cures.

"Honeys, I love you both, but I am afraid I don't have enough faith. It does take faith, you know, as well as herb and vitamins to beat cancer. Maybe I can use both medical and natural remedies. I feel I would have the best chances for a cure that way."

The girls agreed and we sat down to go over the information they had brought.

We discussed each of the vitamins I was going to be taking and what value and purpose they would serve.

The first thing we discussed was to eat organic as much as possible and to eat unprocessed foods. Unprocessed foods are whole foods with nothing added or nothing taken away. Additives to our food serve several different purposes. Some are to extend shelve life, others are to make them more appealing by adding artificial color, texture, or taste. Some additives are natural such as sugar and others such as aspartame (artificial sweetener) are synthetic. Additives add little or no nutritional value to our foods. They can prove to be harmful. Additives thought safe in the past are now label as unhealthily and possible carcinogens such as once widely used saccharin.   The more refined and processed our foods become the less beneficial and less nutritional they are for our bodies.

I had recently made some of these changes in some of our foods but was becoming more aware of the harm to our bodies as I learned more about additives.

The girls had brought a list of vitamins, supplements and foods that would aid me as I began my treatments. These would prove to be a great support for my body's strength to sustain during radiation and chemotherapy.

Mouth Sores Prevention

Among the supplements I began taking was L-Glutamine to help prevent mouth sores from chemotherapy. *I would like to mention here, that this worked wonderfully.* Most of the people I spoke to undergoing chemotherapy, had suffered from mouth sores. None of them had taken L-Glutamine. Tom and I both took it during our treatments and did not get any mouth sores. In addition, a friend of ours diagnosed with pancreatic cancer took the L-Glutamine and he did not get any mouth sores either. It is something you should discuss with your doctor when you start chemotherapy.

Other vitamins and minerals they included were Co-enzyme Q10, which improves cellular oxygenation and supports detoxification. Acidophilus has an antibacterial effect on the body. Flaxseed is an antioxidant, which could aid in the prevention of the cancer from spreading to other parts of your body. Taurine aids with tissue and organ repair and white blood activation. B complex vitamin improves circulation and builds red blood cells and a good daily vitamin that does not contain iron.

They suggested eating Shitake mushrooms, which have a high amount of immune-boosting and anti-tumor properties. I later discovered that there is a supplement, Shitake extract or reishi extract, which will serve the same purpose, especially when you lose your appetite.

I was overwhelmed as they shared this information with me. There seemed to be so much to consider. It was a lot to understand in a short time, but I felt committed to doing all I could to make the radiation and chemotherapy treatments as affective as possible.

They also brought me a copy of *Prescription for Nutritional Healing* by Phyllis A. Balch, CNC and James F. Balch, M.D. It would serve as a good reference for minerals and foods to help promote better health during treatment. I have found this book invaluable as a source to aid with beneficial lifestyle changes.

My daughters' deep concern for my health and healing warmed my heart and gave me strength to face the great unknown ahead of me.

While reviewing all the material they had brought for me, my sister Val and her boyfriend, surprised me with a visit. Val was crying and hugged me and said, "Rita, I love you. I don't want to lose you."

We had grown up in an age where almost everyone diagnosed with cancer had a death sentence. This impacted Val's thinking and manifested her fears that I was going to die. After all, grandma just died from cancer five years ago.

It was strange to sit with my family discussing my health and future cancer treatments. I am still not used to the concept that I have cancer. I wanted my family to feel reassurances that I would become a survivor and one day we could put all of this behind us.

Anal Cancer - Squamous Cell Carcinoma

After everyone left, I decided to learn about my type of cancer. Invasive Squamous cell carcinoma is a mouthful of words.

To begin with, carcinoma is a malignant caner involving the epithelia or skin cells.

23

Epitheliums simply put are skin cells that compose the cells that line cavities and surfaces throughout the body. These surfaces are on the outside skin and inside cavities. Outside skin that can be affected by a carcinoma are face, ears, neck, arms, scalp, and hands. Inside cavities that can be affected by carcinoma are lips, tongue, mouth, esophagus, lungs, and part of the rectum called the anus.

This is a short list of the areas that can be affected by a skin cell cancer, but basically, any surface of the body, inside or out that has skin cells could be affected.

My cancer is squamous cell, which is one of four categories of skin cells. Carcinomas invade the surrounding tissues and organs and may or may not metalized or spread to lymph nodes or other sites. My upcoming test will determine if my cancer has spread to other parts of my body.

That night my journal entry read:

"I am very angry at my doctor. When she discovered the anal lesion, she should have done something about it. Instead, she said it was nothing and not to worry about it. I read that anal lesions are treated as pre-cancerous cells. If she had done something about it at that time, I may have not gotten cancer at all. I had read that If she had taken care of it by cauterization, my odds of developing cancer in that site would have been very close to zero. It makes me very angry at her."

Being told you have cancer is only the beginning of a phase of worry, confusion and an overload of information that is all geared toward recovery and survival from this awful disease called cancer.

I worried about the impact my diagnosis had on my family, especially my children and my husband   "In sickness and health" became primary to our relationship when we, as a couple, had to deal with three words that ultimately changed our lives together, forever.

"You have cancer". Those three little words will set you upon a path of doctors, tests, treatments, and extreme emotions that may become overwhelming at times, and you may feel all alone in your thoughts and feelings.

I remember thinking to myself, after my diagnoses, that I could handle anything that came my way. I had my husband, family and friends for support and felt well-armed for any situation that arouse. Once my journey through cancer began, I realized I was not as well prepared as I had thought.

The idea of having this horrible thing growing inside of me made me shiver. I knew that most people diagnosed with cancer usually turn to the internet to find out more information, but I had no interest in knowing more. I just wanted to go to the doctor and take it from there. I was not ready to deal with it, not just yet, not at the moment. Tomorrow I would deal with it.

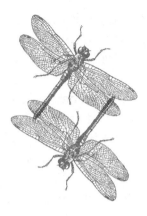

CHAPTER 3 - RITA'S TESTS AND TREATMENT REPARATIONS

Tuesday, September 7, 2004
CT Exam

My CT was scheduled at the local hospital. I have had a CT before, but not with contrast medium. Contrast medium is a dye solution containing iodine given through an IV. The purpose of contrast is to outline organs and soft tissue, making it easier to identify if cancer is present in other locations.

CT or CAT scan is a Computer Axial Tomographic Examination. The CT exam uses numerous x-ray beams plus a set of electronic x-ray detectors, which rotate around your body, measuring the amount of radiation being absorbed by your body. This process produces a series of pictures or sections of your body in a two dimensional cross- section image. Once studied, these cross-sections determine the exact location of a tumor and if it has spread to other parts of the body.

Before going to the radiation department, my first stop was the blood lab. The contrast used for the CT is very strenuous on the kidneys as they filter it out of the body. The blood test is to determine if my kidneys were healthy enough for the contrast, so my creatine level had to be checked. My creatinine and

GFR levels were normal, and I was cleared for my CT.

Creatinine is produced from creatine a molecule of major importance for energy production in muscles. High levels may be a warning of kidney malfunction or failure.

A smile emerged across my face as I entered the testing room. All along the ceiling edge and up and down the walls were paths of paw prints. Like kitten paw prints. Then I realized that people often referred to a CT as a CAT scan. I was impressed by the creativity.

After changing into a gown, I was instructed to lie on a low cloth covered table. The tabletop was on rollers allowing the table to be moved into and out of the waiting CT machine.

Everyone was very friendly and helpful. I lay onto the table and an IV was put into my arm to administer the contrast. I was given instructions to lie as quite as possible and forewarned about a strange sensation I may get from the IV contrast solution.

After the first scan without the contrast was complete, a second scan using the contrast was done. As the contrast liquid entered my body the first sensation was a warm feeling across my face and shoulders. This was followed by a heavy pressure in my chest with a slight burning feeling. I could feel the liquid travel down my body, over my abdomen and bladder and down to my toes. As the pressure of the contrast passed over my bladder, it created the feeling that I had just peed, even though I had not.

I was told to drink plenty of water to flush the contrast dye from my system as quickly as possible. As I had mentioned, contrast is hard on the kidneys. Tom took me home and I slept the rest of the afternoon.

I spent the next few days contemplating my situation. I realized that it was difficult for my family and friends to take the news about my cancer. What could anyone say? It was like being hit in the gut. What can they say?

Anal Ultrasound

Wednesday, September 8, 2004

As the day began, I had no idea how much stress and pressure had built up inside of me. My son, Phillip, took the day off from work so he could go to the two appointments I had scheduled. The first appointment was for an anal ultrasound and the second one was to meet with a radiation oncologist.

What a crazy and exhausting day it became. I already had to begin the day by doing two enemas prior to leaving the house.

The craziness continued, as we got lost in Minneapolis while looking for the hotel where the Pelvic Floor Disorders Seminar was being held. I called the contact number I had been given and asked for further directions. As I parked along the side of the road to make the call, I began to cry. The stress I had been suppressing came to the surface all at once.

Phillip voice was calm and comforting.

"Calm down mom, it will be alright. They will wait for you."

I dried my tears and together we trudged forward. We finally found the hotel, but due to construction, could not find the entrance to the parking ramp. Hidden behind construction equipment the entrance evaded us. Through some degree of endurance, the entrance was finally found, and we were already fifteen minutes late. I began to stress that they would not take me because I was so late.

My panic was unwarranted. Warm greetings met me as I entered the registration area. After completing a history questionnaire of my symptoms and diagnosis, I went to a room where I changed into a gown. Phillip went to another room to wait.

After changing my clothes, we went to a temporary procedure room, and I noticed that there were eight people in the room as I entered it. Everyone was incredibly careful of my modesty and did their best not to expose any more of my personal parts then was necessary for the procedure.

A nurse always stayed at my side, talking to me, and offering me reassurance as the procedure proceeded. I had no idea what to expect. The appointment came up so fast I did not take the time to research what an anal ultra-sound involved.

I lay on my left side with my backside still covered by a sheet. The doctor came in the room and introduced himself. I thought he was great. His voice was very soft and calming. He explained each step of the procedure, both for my sake and that of the 250 doctors viewing from another room via the closed-circuit monitor. He placed a deflated balloon up my rectum and then inflated it. This was to keep the "stuff" in my colon so it could not come out during the exam.

A lubricated probe was then inserted inside my rectum to view the tumor in my anal area, displaying the results on a closed-circuit TV, while the findings were also being recorded. The ultrasound waves bounce off the different tissues allowing healthy, normal tissue as well as defective, abnormal tissues to be seen. It was uncomfortable with some cramping. I tried to breathe slowly and think about my family to remove myself from the immediate awareness of what was happening. The doctor kept asking me if I was doing well. I assured him I was.

As he did the exam, he explained his findings, describing the tumor's location, consistency, and size. What I remember is that the tumor was 4 cm. He also said it was T2N0. I later found out the staging for anal cancer uses letters and numbers to identify its size and stage. T2 meant that my tumor was more than 2 cm and less than 5 cm and that it was a stage I tumor. The N0 meant that I had no regional lymph node metastasis.

A woman using a phone communicated with the doctors in the other room while the exam continued. One question that was asked was a concern that the tumor was touching my urethra. The doctor moved the scope around to take a better look at the area. He said he believed that it was shadowing and not the tumor. At that point, I became more aware that there were 250 people looking at my backside and more. I became a little anxious at that point. The attending nurse once again offered me reassurance. It helped.

The doctor continued the exam relaying additional medical information. I was relieved when the exam was over. I really wanted to get out of there.

Phillip greeted me after the test.

"How are you doing?" he asked.

"I am fine, but I didn't care to much for the test. I am glad it is over, now we have to get to St. Paul."

Radiology

Phillip and I managed to find our way across to St. Paul and the hospital, of which the radiology department facilities and cancer center were within the hospital.

The receptionist took all my pertinent information, insurance and medical card and explained their billing policies. Most of that information went over my head, as I was not really listening. I had too many other things on my mind to concentrate on her words. Phillip, of course, managed to get it all and explained it to me later.

The next step was to provide my personal and medical history. This included any medications or supplements I was taking. The radiology nurse, Donnie, took my medical history, of which I was tired of repeating. She was very kind, and I liked her from the start. Then we waited and waited.

Phillip was being such a trooper all day and I was glad he was with me. As we waited for the doctor to talk with us, my head was reeling from the swiftness of the activities I had participated in over the past week. There was so much information to digest that I was afraid I would miss something important. Phillip's presence proved invaluable, because so much information was given, that in my frame of mind, I missed much of it. Phillip relayed the information to me later after we got home, and I was somewhat settled.

It is especially important to have someone with you at tests and doctor visits. Always carry a notebook to write down questions you want to ask, test information and concerns. I think this is important. The same notebook can be useful for writing answers to these questions and other important information. If I were at this appointment alone, I would have brought a tape recorder because I know I would have missed a lot of information.

I watched Dr. B. as he entered the room. I had seen so many new faces this past week and my intuition about people was in overdrive. So many questions were going through my head as he began to talk. Does this doctor really know what he is doing? Will he really make the right medical choices for me? Can I trust him?

Radiation Oncologist

A Radiation Oncologist is a doctor who specializes in the treatment of cancer patients with the use of radiation therapy. Diagnostic imaging such as an x-ray, ultrasound, MRI (Magnetic Resonance Imaging), and a CT scan are used to help diagnose the disease. With this information, the doctor then develops a plan of treatment that will be the most successful for each patient.

A patient may be treated with either external beam radiation or internal radiation, which is also known as Brachytherapy. Brachytherapy is a radiation source placed next to or into the area requiring treatment.

My treatment would be an external beam radiation.

Dr. B. was soft spoken and relaxed. He was not hurried and was honest about my cancer and prognosis. To my peace of mind, he began on a somewhat positive note.

He explained that if I had this cancer ten years ago the only choice I would have had, was to do surgery, remove the cancer and surrounding areas and insert a colostomy bag. I could feel myself cringe at that thought. He continued to explain that medical treatment for my type of cancer had advanced considerably, and they could now treat the cancerous area without surgery.

He asked some questions about my personal life. After I answered his questions, he asked how my cancer was suspected.

I explained to him how my personal doctor had seen a lesion in the region a few years ago while doing a flexi exam and did nothing about it. In fact, she told me it was nothing and to not worry about it.

I further explained that she had been treating me for a bleeding hemorrhoid for the past two years. I then explained that I did a self-exam and told my doctor I wanted more follow up because I did not believe it was a hemorrhoid. That led to the colonoscopy and ultimately to his office.

The exam results from the anal ultra-sound had arrived and Dr. B. carefully explained them to us. From this information, he was able to describe the size and location of the tumor. He was also able to decide how they were going to treat it with radiation. I would receive 29 doses of front and back pelvic radiation. The doses would increase slightly with each treatment and the treatments would be five times per week for seven and one-half weeks.

Of course, this information did not mean much to me at the time. The impact of those treatments could not have been perceived by me, because I could never had imagined the body could endure the degree of abuse my body was about to receive.

One thing that did stand out and gave me hope was his prognosis of my treatment, which was 85% chance of a cure. It seemed like a high number, and it gave me hope. He also assured me that I would not become radioactive and that contact with other people was not an issue.

He further explained that my cancer was Squamous cell carcinoma of the anal canal. Since the cancer did not invade my lymph nodes, it improved my chances for a cure. It also greatly reduced my chances of cancer metastases to another area of my body.

The hours that followed were filled with more history, tests, and information. This process is called simulation. Again, the information was so overwhelming I continued to be grateful for Phillip's presence.

They did a CT to determine the exact location of the tumor. The radiation therapists were patience and kind. They explained each step to me, as it happened, and the value of what they were doing.

After pinpointing the tumor's exact location, two small "dot" tattoos were put on either side of my hips. The therapist explained the use of the dots were to assure accuracy of the radiation and are used to line up the radiation machine on the same location for each treatment to radiate only the area necessary for treatment.

Radiation Therapy

Radiation therapy uses high doses of radiation to kill cancer cells to prevent them from dividing and continued growth. The radiation machine used to treat cancer differs from those used for an x-ray. This type of radiation uses radioactive substances and that are aimed specifically at the tumor. Unfortunately, the normal cells surrounding the cancerous tumor are also destroyed. Most of the normal cells destroyed during treatment do recover in most cases.

Therefore, the tattoo dots I received over the area to be treated become so important in the delivering of the radiation to the exact area being treated, to help limit damage to the surrounding tissue as much as possible.

After I was tattooed, the nurse, Donnie, took us into an exam room and talked to us about the side effects of radiation treatment. It is difficult to imagine the extent of the side effects and skin damage my body was about to go through. I had never experienced the degree of damage that my body was about to receive, so my imagination could not perceive the information I was receiving.

She further explained that I would have hair loss at the area of radiation and may experience appetite loss, nausea, diarrhea, and fatigue.

I could hear her voice as she spoke, but they were just words. My head whirled and my brain seemed to ache. I could hear her saying things, such as the main side effect I would have would be skin irritation to the radiated area consisting of the front and back pelvic areas. I would also eventually develop painful urination and bowel movements. Donnie emphasized the importance of daily care of this area.

Daily care would consist of a twenty-minute tub soak at first and as the treatment continued as often as five times per day. This was to provide moisture to the area, and cleanliness to prevent infection. She provided me with a high moisturizing salve, Aquaphor and recommend I begin its use right away. She also explained I might begin experiencing urination pain by the end of the first week or the beginning to the second week. She said the pain would be like that of a severe bladder infection. As the information came forth, my head began to spin. Once again, there was too much information, too soon. I decided that I would not try to take all this information in right now and would rely on the printed materials she provided for us.

We did not discuss any permanent side effects that may result from radiation treatment, only the side effects during treatments. I was not aware of the possibility that permanent side effects even existed. This would have been a good time to ask. Many treatments do not have permanent, after treatment, side effects but other treatments do. If you want to be fully informed, it is a good thing to discuss with both your oncologists and radiologist.

When faced with a decision to treat my caner or not, I do not know if permanent post-treatment side effects would have influenced my decision but knowing as much as I could about my treatment and future after treatment would have provided a clearer sense of being fully informed about my options.

My treatment plan also included chemotherapy. Radiation is used to shrink the tumor thus helping the effectiveness of the chemotherapy treatments. I would start my radiation therapy either Monday or Tuesday. I had to meet with Dr. H. first.

I left armed with booklets about radiation, nutrition during treatment and how to handle side effects.

When we arrived home, Phillip and I sat down with Tom and we explained the results of the day with him. He was encouraged by Dr. B.'s 85% chance of a cure. We all were. We shared the booklets with Tom about the treatment, side effects and nutritional needs during treatment. At this point I just wanted to go to sleep and forget about the journey ahead of me.

That night my journal entry was a brief recap of my feelings of the day.

"I'm getting used to knowing I have cancer. I don't like it, but I guess I realize it is a reality and it is happening to me. I don't have the whole picture yet. I may not be as accepting when I do. I also have not started treatment. I am afraid of being sick. My hair will grow back, and I've always wanted to wear hats. I am praying for the best possible news at this point.

I realized I am overwhelmed with it all. I am grateful for my family's support and the comfort in knowing I am not alone."

Clinical Studies
Friday, September 10, 2004

I had an appointment with the clinical studies nurse to discuss the possibility of participating in clinical studies using a treatment that was experimental for anal cancer. Dr. H. had asked me if I would be interested. The appointment was to inform me of the study. If I did enter one, I would receive either the recommended cancer drug treatment of Mitomycin C and 5-FU (5-Fluorouracil) or another cancer drug, Cisplatin. As a participant of the study, I would not know which treatment was being used. It sounded interesting and I decided to consider it. The success rate for the Mitomycin C and 5-FU were good, but the study was to determine if the Cisplatin might be more successful.

The clinical trials nurse provided me with all types of information including the trial schedule of treatments, the support system during treatment and detailed descriptions of each drug. All this information was more than I could absorb.

I took the information home to discuss it with Tom and get his opinion on it all.

Later that day I got my haircut. It was not certain if I

would lose my hair during treatment because at this point, I was not sure if I would be in the study or not. The odds of losing my hair while using the Mitomycin-C and 5-FU were very low, but still existed. The odds of losing my hair while using Cisplatin were very high. Since I did not want to go through a patchy hair loss if I did lose my hair, I decided to get it cut short right now. Shorter hair is so much easier to care for as well. I was anxious to get the process started because I wanted to get the whole thing over with and done.

That night Tom and I met my sister, Lindalee, and her husband, Jeff, at a local restaurant. They surprised me with very thoughtful gifts. One gift was a backpack with rollers and a pull handle.

An affectionate hug accompanied the gift.

Lindalee explained, "I figured this backpack would come in handy for carrying information, medicines, extra clothes or whatever else you may need to have available at any given time," Lindalee explained.

As I looked inside the bag, to my surprise there was a nightgown with a matching robe in lavender floral pattern. One of my favorite colors is lavender.

After we ordered our food, Lindalee handed me a chart indicating a radiation therapy driving schedule.

I looked at the schedule of drivers.

"We all got together and came up with a driving schedule." Lindalee said with a smile. "You are not going to drive yourself or go through one single day alone."

I was touched by her thoughtfulness and the generosity of the friends and relatives whose names appeared on the schedule. I noticed that my friend, Kathy's name appeared on every Monday. I was surprised by this since Mondays were her day off.

Chemotherapy
Monday, September 13, 2004

My appointment with Dr. H. at cancer center was schedule very early giving me the unpleasant chore of driving from

Baldwin to St. Paul during heavy rush hour traffic. This was incredibly stressful for the city girl who had gone country.

I was anxious to get started with my treatment because I wanted it over. I felt too much time had gone by already. As I sat in the waiting area, I thought about the impact this was having on Tom. He was really taking this hard. I wished he would open up and talk about it, but I knew he did not deal with things that way. I hoped there would be time in the future.

Dr. H. and the clinical trials nurse met with me right away. I expressed my interest in the trials, but explained that our insurance company, a privately based company, would not approve of my participation without pre-authorization. I further explained that the approval, if there was one, would take until next week and I did not want to wait.

Dr. H. agreed with my reasoning.

"OK then, let's get started today," he said.

I was surprised that he wanted me to start right away.

"Oh, but I don't have anyone with me to drive me home."

"Don't worry," he explained, "we'll just start tomorrow. We'll get your PICC line in today."

He explained to me that I would receive the chemotherapy drugs of Mitomycin-C and 5-FU. Chemotherapy can be administered intravenously, by mouth, injections or applied to the skin. The type of drugs I would receive would be given intravenously. I was told I would receive my chemotherapy through an IV called a PICC line. A pump attached to this line would slowly pump the chemotherapy drug into my bloodstream over a period of 5 days, 24 hours per day.

PICC Line

As I entered the room where my PICC line would be put into place, I noticed how white and sanitary everything was. Two nurses introduced themselves as they instructed me to lay on the table. I received an explanation of how the procedure would go.

A PICC stands for Peripherally Inserted Venous Catheter

also called a PIC line. An intravenous catheter is inserted through the skin and into a vein in the arm just above the elbow. The catheter tube is long and thin and is advanced through the vein until the tip of it is near the heart.

My height was measured and after calculations, it was determined how long the line should be, so it ended just near my heart on the left side.

After sterilizing my left arm, a shot was injected near the sight of the line entry, to numb the area. The procedure did not hurt except the initial prick to numb the area the catheter line would be inserted. I did not watch. I talked about things that made me feel good, such as my children and my love of writing. Before I knew it, we were done.

After the line was in place, I was sent to x-ray to determine that the location of the line was indeed correct. I could feel the tube inside of me near my heart and it left me with a feeling of uneasiness. It did not hurt, but it symbolized a treatment that I was apprehensive to receive. The x-ray confirmed the correct location.

My first radiation treatment would begin tomorrow followed by the start of my chemotherapy. I felt bewildered at the thought of the upcoming weeks ahead but felt that I was ready to begin.

As I walked out to my car, I realized that there were more decisions to make about treatment than I had thought possible. The tremendous amount of information that I was given to understand, and the swiftness at which it is presented, added more aspects to the decision-making process of treatments. It is all happening so close together. I took a deep breath because I knew that all of this was only the tip of the iceberg.

Once I got home, I attempted to find additional information about my cancer on the internet, but it was more difficult than I thought it would be. As I started looking up information on cancer, I felt OK with it. However, the more I looked, the less I wanted to know. It just made me cry.

I wanted to pretend I did not have cancer. I told myself I

was just going through the process because the doctors wanted me to. It was as though it did not matter if I had therapy or not. It would not affect my life at all. I knew I was wrong. I have this "thing" growing inside of me and the sooner I got started with the process, the sooner it would stop growing.

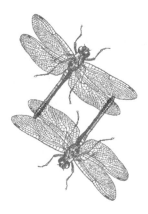

CHAPTER 4 - RITA'S TREAMENTS   BEGIN

Tuesday, September 14

My sister Val, offered to take me for the start of my chemotherapy treatment. When she arrived at my house, I could tell she had been crying.

"What's the matter?" I asked.

"I am so very worried about you. I am afraid of all the things you will have to go through beat your cancer." She said.

I gave her a hug.

"I am going to do very well. I am relatively healthy and strong, and I have all this love and support. How could I not do well?"

Val mustered a smile.

"I guess you're right, but I am still concerned."

I did not have the heart to tell her that I was as anxious about the day ahead as much as she.

Radiation Begins

Once we arrived at radiation center, I was asked to sign a consent form and once again talked about the possible side effects of pelvic radiation. I changed into a gown, removing my entire lower half clothing, and was led into the treatment room.

It was a large room with a gurney style bed in the center. Above the bed, there was a large machine, which reminded me of a camera. My sister Val went into another room with one of the radiation therapists. There was a closed-circuit camera where Val could watch the procedure.

One of the female radiation therapists lined up my hips with my tattoo dots. She then placed a wedge under my knees to elevate them and then she placed a rubber ring around my ankles. The ring was to prevent me from dropping my feet apart causing undesired movement.

I felt apprehensive.

"It's important that you do not move while we do the radiation." She explained.

The therapists were wonderful and patient as they attempted to ease my bewilderment of the whole procedure. As I looked at the ceiling, to my surprise, a soothing picture of a dock over-looking a beautiful lake, greeted my eyes. The picture took the place of a light panel, so the light behind shown through and made the picture more inviting.

The two therapists left the room and a few seconds later spoke to me over a speaker.

"We are going to start now, so stay as still as you can."

The machine hovered above my pelvic area. As I counted, it came to a total of 12 seconds. I began treatment with only front radiation. In a few days, it would become both front and back. As I soon learned, the duration would increase by seconds each day of treatment. I would also learn how damaging radiation would be on both inside and outside tissue.

Treatment went quickly, which surprised me. We then found our way to the cancer center. Chemotherapy would prove to be a long day.

After registering, we went to a private room where I would receive my chemotherapy.

My sister continued her crying off and on all morning. She was more apprehensive and concerned then I was.

"Val don't cry. I will beat this, and things will be just fine."

41

I hugged her to re-enforce my promise.

"I know, but I hate to see you go through all of this. It just doesn't seem fair."

I smiled, "Fair has nothing to do with it. It is what it is, and we just have to do whatever it takes to fix."

Start of Chemotherapy

She dried her tears as the chemotherapy nurse came into the room completely covered by protective clothing and gloves. She explained to us that the chemotherapy drugs are very toxic and contact with her skin as well as mine had to be avoided. This of course created a concern for me about how toxic these drugs were. I was aware of how damaging they are to both healthy cells and cancerous cells. The nurse's attire just re-emphasized this fact.

Before she administered each chemotherapy drug, the nurse explained each step and each drug as we went. She began by flushing my PICC line and changing the dressing. I was given lots of water to drink. The nurse took a syringe full of a blue liquid and attached it to the PICC line. She explained that it was the Mitomycin-C. She very slowly put it into the PICC line, and I watched as the syringe emptied. There was a second syringe. She added it slowly into the PICC line. There was no pain as the deep blue liquid entered my veins.

CADD Infusion Pump (Computerized Ambulatory Delivery Device)

I was given more water to drink. The time had come for the 5-FU (5-Fluorourscil). This is the drug that would be administered via the pump. It would start today and continue twenty-four hours per day until Saturday.

The chemotherapy drug is put into a plastic cassette that fits into the pump. The pump then fits into a bag that hangs from your shoulder. The chemotherapy drug is infused into the blood stream through the pump.

The nurse began by explaining how the pump worked

and what to watch out for as far as possible problems. As I looked at the pump she was holding, I became anxious. My head was so full of new information and terms I had never heard before that taking in even more information seemed almost impossible. The pump made me nervous.

At this point, I expressed my concern about nausea. I explained to her that I become very nauseous easily with most medications and flying. She said I would be given a medication, Zofran, which has proven to be remarkably effective on nausea during chemotherapy.

She continued to show me how the pump operated, how to change the batteries if needed, and how to turn the pump off in case of an emergency. I had no clue what type of emergency that could be, but I listened, just in case.

After I felt more comfortable about the use of the pump, the nurse decided it was time to start it. She gave me the Zofran and more water and turned the pump on. She asked if I felt any pain or discomfort at the site of the PICC line and I told her I did not. I sat there for another hour and since things were going well, she said I could go home.

Armed with yet more handfuls of printed material about cancer treatment, and the pump hanging from a strap on my shoulder, my sister and I headed for home.

Wednesday, September 15, 2004

I was surprised at how great I felt, almost high. The Zofran was working well, and I felt no nausea at all. I was not tired like I had expected. Sleeping was a little difficult. I had to keep track of my IV line and the pump. I had to remember that it was a part of me when I got out of bed to go to the bathroom. Waking up from sleep and having to remember something that is not a normal part of life can be difficult. I also found it difficult to get dressed with the IV line and the pump attached to me. It was very frustrating.

To my surprise, I was not hungry and had to force myself to eat. It took a lot of concentration to eat just one-half of a banana and one-half can of a nutritional drink. I drank my coffee, watered down.

Today was Tom's turn to drive me to my radiation therapy. He went to work in the morning and returned home in time for my appointment at ten o'clock, which would be my permanent appointment time each day.

As Tom and I drove to St Paul, I felt a need to talk with Tom about my treatments.

"The radiation isn't as bad as I thought," I said.

"That's good," he said, "I hate to see you going through all of this, but if this is what it takes to get rid of it, then we can handle it togetgher."

At this point, he seemed as though he did not want to talk about it anymore, so I let it go.

The treatment went quickly and after Tom brought me home, he made us lunch.

"I am not going back to work until you eat something." Tom said.

I remember thinking about how much of a sweetie he was and how much he really loved me. I thought how much I loved him as well.

After I had eaten enough to satisfy Tom, he returned to work. I decided I would take a nap, but could not, because I still felt intimidated by the IV line and pump. I worried that something would go wrong with the pump. I worried that I would pull the line out. I decided to spend this restless time doing some reading about how a person acquired cancer.

Brief Understanding the Cancer Cell

Currently, most of my first thoughts about having cancer were an overwhelming surge of guilt. What had I done wrong to have cancer? Was the cancer a punishment for some wrong I had done earlier in my life? Was it the result of not taking care of my body? Was it from being a smoker?

After my cancer diagnosis, feelings of guilt were entwined with fear, uncertainties, anger, and confusion. I felt guilty that I had not pursued the symptoms and difficulties I had been experiencing for over a year. I felt guilty that I had not been more persistent with my doctor to find the real cause of my symptoms. Anger at my doctor for not doing a follow up on the lesion she had seen years earlier.

My guilt was also coupled with the guilt of spending so much money on health costs. To ease this pain, I asked myself; "Would I spend this money on my husband or children if they got cancer?" My answer was an undeniable, "Yes".

This answer did help to ease some of the financial guilt, but not the guilt of blame I had placed upon me. All these thoughts were running through my mind. I wanted a better understanding of how a healthy human cell could go so terribly wrong as to become cancerous.

Through my reading, I discovered the development of cancer within the human body was not as simple and easy as I had previously believed. Human cells are complicated and required several conditions to become cancerous. It is not as simple as "I did this or that and got cancer." We do not get cancer. We develop cancer from our own bodies based on many factors that caused a healthy cell to become cancerous.

Every cell in the human body reproduces itself to maintain health in the human body. Cells replace themselves if they become damaged such as a scratch, cut or burn on the skin. Cells replace themselves when they become old. There is a gene within each cell, DNA, that has the blueprint to tell the cell how to make an exact copy if itself.

During continued and repeated replacement, occasionally, cells mutate. This means that they are not an exact duplication of the cell they are meant to replace. The gene within the cell tells the mutated cell to die.

If for some reason the gene within the cell is not doing its job, the immune system takes over. The immune system now tells the mutated or unhealthy cell to die. A healthy immune system continually monitors cell reproduction to maintain and protect the balance of healthy cells within our bodies.

Of course, cell reproduction is much more complicated

and involved then how I am presenting it. Please accept my explanation as a working one designed to help develop an understanding of how cancer develops in the human body.

As I stated earlier, each cell has a control center or blueprint called a gene. When a healthy cell reproduces as a mutation, the gene becomes a precancerous cell. If this cell continues to reproduce unchecked by the immune system, it becomes what is called an oncogene or cancerous. Once this happens, the blueprint that would have told the deformed cell to die is now changed. The oncogene tells the cell to continued reproduction of itself, and not to stop. If the immune system is not healthy enough to control this wild oncogene, it will continue to reproduce and grow into large masses that are known as cancerous growths or tumors. These cells have become immortal. These cells will continue to grow as long the host body, human or animal continues to live.

Many factors influence the reproduction of both healthy and mutated cells. Maintaining a healthy immune system is the best prevention against the development of unwanted, unhealthy cells. From my earlier explanation about cell reproduction, you can understand the vital importance of a healthy immune system.

Other factors that affect the reproduction of muted cells or oncogenes are diet, environment, and habits such as tobacco and alcohol use, viruses, genetics, and emotional health.

The human body reproduces billions of cells each day. The more often cells are reproduced, the higher the risk of mutation. Maintaining a healthy body helps to decrease the chances of producing mutated cells.

High fat foods such as polyunsaturated fats and trans fats promote the growth of free radicals. Free radicals are needed for certain functions of the body, but ones created by high fat content in the body promote the possibly of creating mutation or damage to a healthy cell. For addition information on free radicals, please refer to the book *Prescription for Nutritional Healing* by Phyllis A. Balch, CNC and James F. Balch, M.D., of which I recommended earlier. It has a very good explanation.

The understanding of how important emotional health is to the body is more understood now, than in the past. Stress, depression, and other negative emotional behaviors stress the immune system and weaken its ability to protect our cells.

As I have said, the immune system is vital in the reproduction of healthy cells. This mutation process is more complicated than what I am presenting, but my goal is to help you understand that many factors affect the mutation of a cell. No one cause is to blame and there are no guarantees that you will never be diagnosed with cancer. Understanding this process can help to relieve the overwhelming guilt about developing cancer. As humans, we can only do our best to create a healthy body and cannot control factors that we have no power over.

Cancer Cells and Chemotherapy

Since we understand that cancer cells are not foreign organisms but are reproduced in our own bodies, it is helpful to know how chemotherapy works.

Cancer cells are rapid reproducing cells and chemotherapy drugs are aimed at these fast-growing cells. Many of our natural cells such as hair follicles and gastrointestinal tract and mucus membranes are fast growing cells as well. Since chemotherapy does destroy fast growing cells first, many people may experience hair loss, stomach upset and mouth sores from treatment.

Chemotherapy destroys the DNA of the cancer cell and either kills it right away or weakens it so it cannot reproduce.

Healthy cells can repair themselves more quickly than cancer cells, which allow us to survive the strong toxins of chemotherapy during treatment.

There may be long-term risks associated with chemotherapy. Some of them may be risks to your heart, liver or even the risk of another type of cancer. Be sure to talk to your doctor about these long-term risks. They may not change your mind about treatment, but as I have mentioned, it is nice to know as much as you can.

I found the information I had read interesting and was fascinated by the complex makeup of the human body. The information satisfied my need to develop a better understanding of cancer and treatments.

Thursday, September 16, 2004

"I feel much better today. Yesterday I was tired all day. I managed to load the dishwasher but that was all. I read about Zofran (for nausea) and discovered that it would cause drowsiness until I adjusted to it. I am continuing to use the Aquaphor daily for skin health and I am soaking 20 minutes, once per day. So, for today, anyway, I feel good".

Kathy took the day off so she could drive for me today. Once again, radiation therapy seemed surprising quick. I am noticing however, that I am experienced groin cramps. I was surprised by this since it was only my third radiation treatment.

Kathy remained her happy and bubbly self as she helped me feel more at ease about my situation.

"Let's do lunch," she proclaimed. I thought it was a good idea. We ate Chinese.

"OK," she announced, "Let's go shopping. Pretty soon you will need some dresses to wear, and I just love shopping for dresses."

I was told that within a short time I would no longer be able to wear underwear. Once my skin begins to experience continued damage, fabric against it will progressively become uncomfortable and painful. My only clothing option will become dresses or skirts.

My appreciation for Kathy and her support grows with each day. Her positive attitude and friendship warm my heart and gives me strength. I know that a strong support system is often an important element to a cure. If you were to describe my personality, it would be stubborn and independent. The most common used phrase in my vocabulary is "I can do it myself".

I have always been an independent person, rarely asking for help from anyone. I have been known to have great tenacity.

I got that from my grandmother, Frieda. At eighty years old, she was diagnosed with colon, stomach, and liver cancer. The cancer was quite progressed, so she decided to go to one of the best cancer centers in the country.

My sisters, Sandy and Val took her to the clinic. After she underwent many tests and exams, the doctor entered the room to share his diagnosis and opinion about it.

He told her he was sorry, but the cancer had advanced so there was nothing they could do for her. He told her that she had lived a good, long life, so she should go home and live what time she had left. He told her to go home and live the best she could until she died. He told her she had about six months.

My grandmother and sisters were dumb founded. This doctor was telling her to go home and die. After leaving the hospital, the three of them sat down by the water fountain and cried. When my grandmother finished crying, her words shocked my sisters.

"I'll show that bastard doctor. I am going to go home and fight this. I am not going to just lie down and die. How dare he say that to me?"

My grandmother started chemotherapy with her regular doctor and a local oncologist. My mother was at her side, giving her support and strength whenever she needed it.

A tradition my grandmother had carried on for over sixty years was to bake bread on Thursday so she would have enough to last the week. Her house always smelled so good. On the last Thursday of her life, she was baking bread. She died the next Monday; three years after the doctor had told her to go home and die. She had great tenacity and to this day, I am grateful she had passed it on to me.

There were times during my treatment and recovery that I though about her.

I would tell myself on the days when I felt discourage, "Grandma would be really mad at me if she knew how discouraged I felt. She'll come back down here and kick my butt." Just remembering her and her strength during her long fight with cancer, gave me the strength and faith to continue my fight, and make her proud of me.

Be open to all the support and help you can get. Their strength will become an important element to your cure. Believe me, there will be times when you want to give up. Call on the people within your support system and use their love, care and strength to pick yourself up and go on.

Friday, September 17, 2004

I noticed that my energy level is decreasing, and I am becoming less and less interested in eating. When my daughter Valerie arrived to take me to my fourth radiation treatment, she greeted me with such great love and affection that is gave me strength. She is such a ray of sunshine.

Her concern for my nutritional health became evident when we met with the nutritionist after my treatment. Valerie was fascinated with some of the advice I was given, and she became my main source of nutritional information since her and her twin sister, Rachel, had become exceptionally aware of the importance of nutrition.

They had become vegetarians five years earlier and were two of the healthiest people I knew. I put a lot of my trust in them both.

Before we arrived home, I started to get severe stomach cramps. I knew it was just a matter of time before the radiation treatments would begin to take their toll on my body. I feared I was not ready for the changes I would soon face.

Saturday, September 18, 2004

I noticed that my stomach cramps seemed to be increasing. My bowel movements were very irregular, but I did not have diarrhea yet, which is one possible side effect of pelvic radiation.

I was anxious to get the PICC line out as I found the tape had become very irritating. I had gotten used to the strange sensation on my left side under the skin along the PICC line pathway even though some days it was more annoying than others.

Phillip took me to our local hospital to have the IV removed. Tom was torn between taking me to the hospital or going to the last car show of the year.

We talked about it and I told Tom I wanted him to go to the car show. It was great fun, and I did not want Tom to miss the last car show of the year. He finally gave in and decided to go, especially since Phillip offered to take me to the hospital for the removal of the PICC line.

I was not sure what to expect when we arrived at the hospital. I knew nothing about the IV/chemotherapy department at our local hospital. It is strange how much trust you develop with nurses along the way who have already been caring for you. At our hospital, I did not know the nurse who would care for me today and was nervous.

Once we arrived, we learned that there was not a chemotherapy nurse on duty. I felt a tinge of panic. One of the floor nurses was going to do the procedure of removing the PICC line. I had been given a removal kit when I had received the pump and I brought that with me. It included a container for the proper disposition of the toxic materials that the PICC line and related articles had become.

The nurse was noticeably young and seemed to have no clue of what she was doing. To begin with, it hurt like hell to have the tape removed from the line entrance. My skin was irritated and blistered under the tape. The young nurse continued and seemed unaware of the toxic material she was dealing with. I had to give her warnings about the toxicity and dangers of the chemo drug. I had to help her with the toxic kit. She finally got the idea that she was not taking out just any PICC line. She was a little rough, but got the job done.

I then gave further instructions to help on how to package the disposal kit, including everything for the pump kit so it could be returned. It seemed strange to me that a professional did not know what she was doing. After a little more thought, I realized that she was not a Chemotherapy nurse, and it was as new to her as it was to me.

I was relieved that the line and the pump were gone. I noticed that my lips were dry and wrinkly. I made a mental note to myself that I needed to drink more liquids. I had feelings of general tiredness and some weakness but did not seem to feel as though I was experiencing fatigue. It was hard for me to know for sure what fatigue actually felt like, but believe me, as my treatments continued, I did fully learn to realize the difference between tiredness and fatigue.

When we returned home from the hospital to my surprise, my mom and dad stopped by for a visit. I was tired and did not feel very social, but they had come so far to visit. I sat and visited with them even though I felt a little foggy. My dad gave me a nice box of chocolates and a fluffy white housecoat. They are obviously concerned about my health. It is hard to imagine how they feel. After all, I am their daughter.

Sunday, September 19, 2004

I was awakened rudely this morning with diarrhea, which lasted all day long. I did not know how to stop it. If I had read the information on controlling side effects, I would have known what to do. Be sure to read all the information you are given. It can make a difference.

Tom and I watched the Packer game today. The Packers lost. However, it was fun to watch the game with him. Watching football is one thing that we both enjoy, and shared.

By bedtime, the diarrhea continued, all night and into the morning.

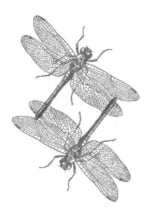

CHAPTER 5 - MANIFESTATION OF RITA'S SIDE EFFECTS

Monday, September 20, 2004

When Kathy arrived at my house to take me to my fifth radiation treatment, she said I looked like hell. I explained to her, that about eight o' clock that morning, I had decided not to eat or drink anything because I was afraid of having the diarrhea on the way to treatment. Because of that decision, I became dehydrated. The left side of my throat, behind my tongue and down in inside of my throat and neck became sore and painful from lack of fluids.

When I arrived at treatment, the nurse suggested that I see the doctor right after the session to discuss the diarrhea and the throat soreness.

The nurse suggested that I use a type of anti-diarrhea product, drink lots or water and a high nutrient drink such as Gatorade. After following these instructions, the diarrhea was under control, my throat pain lessened, and I felt better overall.

The skin on my butt, thighs and vaginal areas were becoming more tender, sore, and painful with each treatment, so Kathy and I decided to buy a sitz bath. A sitz bath is a plastic basin, which is placed into the toilet and filled with water. A water bottle is hung above the sitz and has a clear tube that is inserted into the back of the plastic basin. This tube feeds fresh water in as the old water drains out an opening into the toilet. The sitz did help tremendously and was easier for me to set up then getting in and out of the tub by myself. I used it two times daily for 20 minutes each. I would sit in the tub when Tom was home to help me.

Wednesday, September 22, 2004

I did not have treatment yesterday as the radiation equipment was down. So today will be my sixth radiation treatment. Phillip drove today and was very quiet about the whole thing. Phillip keeps telling me that I am going to be all right and will beat this. I suspect that he tells me this, partially for my sake. Also, partially, to convince himself that is it true.

I fight diarrhea everyday now. I have been lucky and making it home before it starts.

Everyone at radiology is impressed with my support system. I am too. I am very grateful. I realize how important it is to have a support system to make it through all the driving, treatments and continued positive attitude that I will survive.

It is still difficult for me to accept so much help from other people. I have been so independent all my life. I guess it makes me feel so vulnerable. No one wants to feel vulnerable, but the fact is, at a time like this, I am vulnerable. Stress, concern, and physical damage to my body weaken my endurance and help from others becomes very important to recovery. Just having someone to share my concerns and fears with is important as well.

Thursday, September 23, 2004

Tom drove me to my seventh radiation treatment today. The therapists let him in the control room so he could watch the process. I remember the first day I had treatment, I was very apprehensive. As I counted the time in seconds, I discovered that the treatments indeed were getting longer each day. I now received treatment first from the top of my pelvis and then the machine rotated underneath me, and I received the treatment to the back of my pelvis.

Today we barely made it to Hudson, about fifteen minutes, before I had to run into a gas station. I forgot to take some anti-diarrhea medication after treatment, which helps me to make it all the way home.

Tom made sure I ate some lunch and then went back to work. I slept most of the day until he came home. He scrubbed out the tub, filled it for me, and then helped into it so I could do my twenty-minute soak. I missed my afternoon sitz because I was so tired.

I slept some more after that. I seemed to be feeling tired more often these days. I have been sleeping on the couch more and more at night. I feel more comfortable sleeping alone. I miss sleeping with Tom and he misses me.

I noticed that Tom had been coughing a lot lately, so I asked him to go to the doctor and get it checked out. I remember adding that I was concerned that he may have picked up something and I was afraid of catching it. I felt very vulnerable about germs and such lately. He told me he would get it checked out. When he did go to the doctor, he was told the coughing was from his blood pressure medication. It seemed strange that it suddenly caused coughing as he had been on it for years.

Friday, September 24, 2004

My daughter Val drove again today for my eighth radiation treatment. The week went fast. My arm is healing well and looking much better. The blisters are gone and so is the pain. Everyone at treatment were happy to see Val again as she was well liked by all of them.   As time went by in my treatment, eating became more and more difficult each day. My main problem with eating was a loss of appetite. I was told that both chemotherapy and radiation might affect appetite.

After treatment, we went shopping for jewelry making supplies for Val. She had some projects going and needed some materials to finish. It was nice spending the day with her. Since the girls have been at college, I did not see them as much and really missed them. I was very appreciative to Val for taking time away from classes to be a part of my support system.

Saturday, September 25, 2004

No treatment today but I have severe stomach cramps. The crack in my butt is getting extremely sore. I have had insomnia for two days now and I cannot even take naps. I feel very tired, but I cannot sleep. I am having more difficulty with urination pain. It hurts so much I find myself clenching me teeth. The pain is ten times worse than a bladder infection.

Sunday, September 26, 2004

No treatment today and the Packers lost. I have found that keeping myself interested in the things I value, helps me to get through the tough days that seem difficult to handle.

Monday, September 27, 2004

Kathy arrived to take me to my ninth radiation treatment. I was amazed at how quickly treatment went, even though I know it was getting longer each day.

We stopped and ate Chinese food today. I really enjoy Chinese food so eating went well today. After arriving home, I slept for the afternoon. I am soaking two times per day now. I find the effectiveness of the sitz bath not as beneficial as it was at first. It is getting uncomfortable to sit on the hard plastic. I am still using it when no one is home to help me with my bath.

Tom cleaned the tub when he got home and got my soak ready. While I was soaking, he brought a TV into the bathroom so I could watch it as I soaked. He takes such good care of me. I am soaking for about thirty minutes. It does make a difference if I miss it. I am also using the moisturizing cream called Aquaphor after each soak. It soothes and protects the damaged skin and promotes healing as well. I cannot imagine how awful my skin would be without it. It is getting so sore to the touch and turning a dark brown.

Tuesday, September 28, 2004

As my sister, Val, arrived to take me to my tenth radiation treatment, she surprised me with a gift of two cute hats today. It was thoughtful of her, but it has been decided that I am not going to lose my hair with this chemo drug. I have decided to keep my hair short though, as it is easier to take care of. I will donate the hats to the chemo department at local hospital.

Wednesday, September 29, 2008

As Phillip drove me to my eleventh radiation treatment, he is still very quiet about it all. After treatment today, the nurse, Donnie asked me if I was interested in having contact from a woman, Gloria, who had the same cancer, anal cancer, as I did. She explained that I had taken over her time slot for radiation treatments. I told her I would be interested and asked her to give the woman my number.

The burning with urination is markedly worse. Bowel movements are quite painful as well and increasingly worse. It even hurts when I am not going to the bathroom. I have received a few suggestions to help ease the pain. These include peeing in the sitz bath or spraying my body with a spray bottle of water. These hints do not seem to work for me.

I found that holding a large bladder control pad against myself when I urinate, works best. I remove it quickly when I am done. It seems the liquid passes into the pad and stays off my skin, so it does not burn as much.

I have increased my tub soaking to three times per day. I soak before Tom leaves for work, again when he gets home and a third time before bed. The water really helps to ease the soreness and pain in my vaginal and rectal areas.

Thursday, September 30, 2004

My niece, Julia drove to my twelfth treatment today. She lives fifty miles from my house. After she took me to the cities and back to my house, she still had to drive home. Lots of love to Julia. The love and support from family and friends has become as important to my recovery and survival as the treatments themselves.

Friday, October 1, 2004

My sister Lindalee drove me to my thirteenth treatment today. She lives further away than Julia. I once again feel very blessed to have such a supportive family. I am impressed at the love and kindness I have been blessed to have. After radiation treatment, she took me to a local hospital for my mammogram. She was wearing tennis shoes with bright hot pink laces. October is Breast Cancer awareness month, and she was showing her support.

Saturday, October 2, 2004

Gloria, the woman Donnie had told me about at radiation therapy, called me today. She lies in Afton, Minnesota. It was inspiring to talk with her. She is coming for a visit on Wednesday. I was looking forward to visiting with her. I am hoping for conversations with her that will offer insight and strength a support group may have offered.

There were cancer support groups at the hospital where I receive radiation, but I don't want to impose any further on all the people who are presently driving me to treatments, to take me to one.

Monday, October 4, 2004

It is another Monday and Kathy drove me to my fourteenth radiation treatment today. It is getting more and more difficult to get up on the treatment table. Partially because of the pain I feel when my bottom sits on the table and partially because I am feeling more tired every day. I no longer wear any underwear either. Fabric against my skin is painful, so I have begun to wear just dresses and skirts.

Tuesday, October 5, 2004

My sister Val drove today for my fifteenth radiation treatment. She comes even further then my sister Lindalee. When people do so much for you, you wonder how you will ever be able to repay them. I know none of them is doing it for reward and I think they will never know how important their support is to me.

Wednesday, October 6, 2004

Tom drove today, sixteenth treatment. I like it when Tom can drive so we can spend important time together. I am starting to have more difficulty sitting and peeing is getting much more painful. I am also tired most of the time lately.

After Tom returned to work, Gloria, the cancer patient

Donnie told me about, came for a visit. Since she had the same cancer in the same place with the same treatments, I could so fully relate to her. Her progress gave me a point to understand what I was in for and how I may likely progress. She is still recovering but making good progress. Being able to relate to another human being about your state of mind and body is so important. It gives strength and offers hope.

Thursday, October 7, 2004

My niece Christina, who lives near my sister Lindalee, came to take me to treatment today, but her daughter began throwing up on their way over. I told Christina to take her home and I would find someone else to drive me. She felt badly about it, but I felt badly that her daughter was sick and knew she needed to go home. Thank goodness, a friend of mine, Sue, who was on a back-up list, was able to drive.

Friday, October 8, 2004

My daughter, Val, drove today. She had a lot of fun visiting with the radiation therapists today. It is refreshing to see the wonderful, outgoing personality of hers. Her attitude about life is so positive and inspiring as well. I feel great pride when I think of my children and the fabulous adults they have become.

My sister Sandy is coming from Oregon tomorrow. I am looking forward to her visit. It was nice of her husband, Larry, to let her come here for a month. It will be nice to have someone around all day. I get so tired and do not feed myself or soak during the day when no one is around. The soak baths are extremely important. Time is going by quickly, so quickly that I am losing track of time.

Saturday, October 9, 2004

Tom and I picked Sandy up from the airport today. Lindalee met us for breakfast. Sandy was exhausted from being up all night since she had taken the overnight flight. Things are starting to get confusing for me now. I feel tired all the time and cannot seem to get enough sleep. I am glad Sandy is here. I am close to her, and her presence is giving that extra boost of endurance I need to get through this whole thing.

Monday, October 11, 2004

Today was my nineteenth radiation treatment and the start of my second chemotherapy treatment. Kathy drove and Sandy came with. Sandy does not drive freeways and Kathy had already volunteered to drive every Monday so that was very helpful.

Today was an exceptionally long day as it was the start of my second chemotherapy treatment. The day started on the wrong foot. It was a holiday, Columbus Day, and the cancer center was on short staff for the day.

I was supposed to get my PICC line at 8:50 a.m., but no one in the department was aware that I needed it. We waited two hours before someone realized what I needed. After my PICC line was in place, I went to radiation for my treatment. After radiation, I had my blood count done. My White cells were 6.8, red cells were 12.5 and platelets were 294,000 all within a healthy range. My creatinine level was normal. I am continuing to use the Zofran and Compazine for nausea. I am finding an upset stomach and vomiting is becoming more of a problem as treatment progresses.

Since it was way after lunch, Sandy begged someone for some soup for me to eat. I was surprised at how well it went down. We waited for a nurse to come and take me to start my chemotherapy.

Finally, a nurse greeted us after my PICC was in and led the three of us to a small room. We managed to all squeeze into the room as the nurse began to explain the procedure to me. I am sure she knew that I was already fully aware of what was going to happen as it was my second session of Chemo, but too much information is better than not enough.

Kathy was apprehensive. I have never seen her that way before. I took some Zofran for the nausea and a full glass of water. This was followed by the first phase of my treatment, which consisted of the two syringes full of Mitomycin C through my PICC line. After the Mitomycin C was completed, my pump with the 5-FU was attached and started.

I think Kathy was more relieved that the procedure was finally over more than I was.

Aside from my bottom being painful and sore, I was in good spirits. It was reassuring to have Sandy staying with us.

I continued my tub soaks three times a day. Sandy was very helpful. She started a chart indicating what medications I needed, when, and how much. She also tracked my nutritional and water intake. She numbered the bottles to make sure I was drinking enough water. Water was important since my skin was being baked at each radiation treatment and losing most of its moisture each time.

Currently, I was on Zofran and Compazine for nausea, and Pyridium to help ease the intense urination and bladder pain, which was increasing daily.

Tuesday, October 12, 2004

My sister Val drove and Sandy came with. The weather had turned cold, and the chemo pump made it impossible to wear a jacket, so I wrapped up in a blanket and used it for warmth.

My buttocks, inside my thighs, rectal and vaginal area were becoming extremely raw and sore by now. I sat on chucks (bladder control flat pad) and set a bladder control pad beneath me as we drove. I took my anti-diarrhea pills and away we went.

We went out for lunch at a local restaurant that made the best potato soup ever. Val bought me some to take home.

Wednesday, Thursday, October 13 and 14, 2004

I do not remember these days very well, as I was becoming less able to tolerate my pain by this time. All attempts to use pain control medication have failed. I am allergic to codeine, which is the base for most pain medications I would otherwise be taking. The Chemotherapy was making me very sick. I throw up a lot and fight nausea all the time. I found the pump very irritating this time. It was serving as a reminder that I was fighting cancer and bothered me more than it ever had.

First Hospitalization

Friday, October 15, 2004

My sister Lindalee and her husband Jeff took me to my twenty-third radiation treatment. They picked Sandy and me up from my house. I was doing pretty well when they picked me up and when we got to radiation treatment. While we were waiting for the PICC line to be removed, I started getting sick, nauseous, and dizzy. My pain level had escalated and the whole world had become a blur. Sandy told the nurse what was happening, so I was put into a private room to wait for Dr. H. to see me.

Dr. H. arrived and checked me over. He indicated that my skin was worsening, but not infected. His biggest concern for me at the time was uncontrolled pain. He asked me if I wanted to go into the hospital. I told him I was confused and did not know what to do. He said he would make the decision for me and put me into the hospital. He mentioned that he wanted me to spend the weekend in the hospital.

Before going up stairs to a hospital floor, the PICC was removed.

I was admitted for uncontrolled pain, nausea, urination pain and extremely damaged/red skin injury. My white count was 6.2, my red count was good at 11.5 and my platelets were within range at 271,000.

PCA (Patient Controlled Analgesia)

The impression I remember about this floor and room was unwelcoming. The halls were dark, and gloomy, and it seemed no one smiled, and people were unpleasant.

I was started on PCA Morphine (Patient Controlled Analgesia). This form of drug administration allows the patient to control the amount they receive. It does have a limit on how often a patient can receive the drug, to avoid the possibly of an overdose.

Dr. H. wanted to discover what doses I could handle. I needed some degree of pain control. Once a successful dose is discovered, I would be sent home on an oral Morphine drug. Tom and Phillip came to the hospital right away. I had a woman doctor, who was impatient and seemingly uncaring. I did not like her from the start. Tom and Sandy did not like her either. She was not compassionate and did not consider my actual condition. All she wanted was for me to go home. I could not understand her thinking. Dr. H. wanted me to stay until Monday, but each time she came in, she asked me if I was ready to go home.

Saturday, October 16, 2004

The same female doctor continued to insist that I go home. She expressed that she felt I had no need to be in the hospital. On her report, she claimed that I agree to go home. That was not the case, but she released me against my will. I was sent home on a prescription of Dilaudid for pain, a very small dose. Tom and Sandy had difficulty finding the correct dose because it was so small, 1 mg. Finally, after checking with three pharmacies who said they did not carry that dose, Tom asked the last one what size they did carry.

The Pharmacist said 2 mg. Tom asked if they sold pill splitters and if cutting one on half would work. The pharmacist said it would work quite well. Finally, a solution was found. All this time of running around, I was lying in the back seat of the car not doing very well. I was so sick and nauseas that I could not stand it. I was dizzy, miserable, and just wanted to get into bed and stop moving. All that could have been avoided if the first pharmacist at the hospital would have just mention they only had 2 mg and came up with the solution that Tom did. I do not remember much else.

Sunday, October 17, 2004

All I remember is feeling very nauseous and dizzy. I did not want to eat but Sandy made sure I drank a nutritional drink and water.

Monday, October 18, 19 2004

Kathy and Sandy took me back to the hospital for my radiation treatment. I got sick at radiation and the nurse, Donnie, felt I should go to the cancer Center and see Dr. H. While we were waiting at the center, everything fell apart. I was vomiting, dizzy, and sick. I barely remember anything as it was all such a blur. Dr. B.'s nurse was instrumental.

She became my guardian angel that day. She stayed with me and helped me through my vomiting. Even when I had nothing left to vomit, she spoke to me gently, told me to relax, and left it go. I was crying and felt so discouraged. Everything hurt and I felt like giving up. Somehow, I found myself in a gown and had no idea when that happened. I barely remember moving through the halls on a gurney and Dr. B.'s nurse being protective of my privacy as we rolled along the hallways. While I was in x-ray, I remember having to go pee while they were doing the test. The tech told me not to worry about and just go. She said she would get me a clean gown.

Second Hospitalization

I barely remember being put into a room. The cancer care floor was full, so I was put in an available room. Shortly thereafter, I remember Sandy and Kathy were there. Again, I did not care for the floor nurses. They appeared to dislike their jobs and had little compassion for the patients. Not only is family support very important, but the attitude of health care people is just as important.

The rest of the day was a blur, Tom came to the hospital so Sandy, and Kathy went home.

After family members left for the night, I do remember asking a nurse to help me apply the Aquaphor to my butt area. The nurse took one look at the damaged skin and said, "I'm not touching that", and left the room. By this time, I was feeling more nausea and dizzy then ever and the whole world seemed to be changing into a dream. I do not even remember if the cream got on my butt or not.

I remember hearing people's voices but not understanding what they were saying and that their voices just boomed in my head, making it ached more than it already did.

When food was brought to me it looked good and smelled good, but I just could not eat. The best way to describe the loss of appetite is, imagine a wonderful holiday dinner and then imagine that you have eaten so much you feel stuffed. You decide to take one more bite, but you chew and chew and no matter how hard you try to swallow that bite, you cannot. That is how it feels to lose your appetite during cancer treatment. The desire to swallow just is not there.

Tuesday, October 19, 2004

Kathy took the week off work so she could bring Sandy to the hospital each day. Kathy later told me that I had been complaining about my pain, so the unlikable woman doctor told her she would give me a suppository for the pain. Kathy was horrified and told the doctor that there was no way she was going to give me a suppository. She explained to this doctor about the radiation treatments and all the tissue damage to the rectal area. The doctor simply relied "Oh" and no longer addressed my pain.

Sandy later told me that my language started to become "colorful". At radiation treatment, I began vomiting again. The nurse at radiation asked me what I was throwing up. I guess I told her I didn't know and didn't f--king care." It was a bad day.

One thing that stood out that day was that the same woman doctor kept asking me if I wanted to go home. It seemed like every time she came in, that was her biggest concern. Not my health, but that I should go home. My pain was still uncontrolled, I was not eating or drinking, I was throwing up all the time, and she wanted me to go home. My sister Sandy took a marker and wrote in huge letters on my daily message board, "SHE IS NOT GOING HOME!"

Wednesday, October 20, 2004

The written message did not seem to impress this doctor, because the first thing she asked me the next morning was if I wanted to go home.

The next thing I remember, was seeing a bag of blood hanging over my head and a nurse putting the tube into my IV. Oh! I was getting a blood transfusion, yet this doctor had wanted me to go home. Tom spoke with Dr. H. and after that, I did not see that doctor again.

Sandy and Kathy arrived shortly after the transfusion

had begun. I am not certain about the duration and amount of the blood I was given, but I do remember asking if I was going to die. I do not know if I got an answer to that question, because my existence had become surreal. I felt as though I had been separated from my family by a sheer curtain, and even though I could see my family, I could not hear them. I was having my own conversation on my side of the curtain, but I am not sure with whom.

I asked again if I was going to die. I felt a presence but there was no answer. Then I said, "I'm not ready yet. Not yet."

About then, the curtain seemed to disappear, and I could see and hear my family again. It was a strange day and a strange experience, but the transfusion brought my red blood cells back to a safe level and I started feeling better. My blood count had dropped to 6.5. Later I found out that eight and below become life and death critical.

Tom's brother Al came by to visit, but I have no memory of his being there. I knew he came because my sister Lindalee put out a book for visitors to sign and leave words of encouragement for me.

Here are a few of those notes. The first one is from my daughter, Val.

"Hey mom. Aunty Lindalee thought it would be fun to keep a journal for you so you can have a reference point when this is all over. I'm sorry I asked you if you were hungry so many times. I know you are very uncomfortable and in a lot of pain. We are all praying for you.
Today we waited for Dr. H. all afternoon and were all amazed at the "micromanagement" and disorganization of the hospital. Don't worry we'll make sure we know what is happening. VAL"

The second entry is from my daughter Rachel.

"Hey mom – It's my first time at the hospital. I knew chemotherapy would be hard on you, but I am not used to you being so vulnerable. All I can remember you been the strong one while I was sick. I will be strong for you. I have been asking questions of all the nurses, interns and assistants that come in to see you. WE are all watching

out for you because we want the best for you. Love you – Rachel".

The next entry was from my brother-in-law, Al.

"Toked yaun hwo – Call if u need anything – your brother-in-law – Al Kasinskas. Waste waun."

It is Sioux and I have no idea what it he said.

The fourth entry was from my sister, Lindalee.

"Hi Rita, It's 4:15 p.m. Wednesday. You are looking better in some ways and not so good in others. I think you are in a tie with dad and Pat in the "how many lines can we put in them" contest. Look forward to your recovery! WE are praying for you. God be merciful. God be graceful. I love you sis! Your oldest sis, Lindalee."

Another thing I do remember is that the nurses did not seem to be concerned if I got my extremely important soak baths. I needed at least four per day. Whenever I asked I about the bath, the nurse would just say, "I'll be back in a while to help you with that", yet no one ever came back. I remember when Tom came to see me, he would wet towels and place them around my raw, dry, damaged skin to help retain some moisture.

Finally, Tom went to my doctor and told him about the lack of concern and the lack of care I was receiving. The next day the head nurse came in and I explained to her the importance of my bath soaking four times per day. It ended up that I received two baths with help per day after that. The other two times I had to walk down the hall to the tub, fill it myself and get in myself. It seemed as though no one felt that all aspects of patient care were in his or her job description.

Thursday October 21, 2004

My skin is deteriorating in conjunction with the radiation treatments, very raw and discolored. The skin is a very dark brown and, in the crevasses, there were pockets of soft white flesh. It hurts to sit, and it hurts to pee. I feel very miserable and want the whole thing to be done with. I remember thinking I did not know how much more I could handle.

After my twenty-seventh radiation treatment I remember being in my hospital room and saying that I did not want to do this anymore. The new doctor I had, a very nice man, prescribed an antidepressant for me.

While Sandy and Kathy were visiting, they set up my soak bath, took me down to the room, and helped me. The nurses still did not seem to care.

I was looking forward to completing my last radiation treatment on Monday. Later that day when Dr. H. came in, the conversation centered on my ability to travel the fifty miles back and forth for my continued radiation treatments. I was at the point where I started vomiting every time I moved around.

Kathy and Sandy had been discussing this very thing. When Dr, H came in, Kathy mentioned to him that every time I was moved either to go to radiation or to go to the bathroom, I began throwing up. She suggested to him that it might be motion sickness.

Dr. H. agreed that it was common for chemotherapy patients to have motion sickness. Dr. H. prescribed a motion sickness patch and I stated having some improvement over the nausea. I still did not want to eat but began taking in more liquids.

The patch also seemed to help me tolerate the morphine that I was taking for pain control. Little improvements feel like large ones, if it improves my ability to handle my continued treatment.

Dr. H. was trying to decide if it would be advisable for me to stay at the hospital until my last treatment on Monday. While discussing this option, he reviewed my treatment records and informed us that I was schedule for three additional "boost" treatments. That meant I would not be done with radiation until Thursday. I began to cry. I cannot even explain how that just broke my heart to think of five more treatments. I wanted to be done.

The idea of traveling back and forth over the next week depressed me because I knew I would be sick from the driving.

Dr. H. explained that he could not justify a hospital stay until Thursday. The best he could do was Sunday.

My sister Val's boyfriend, Rob, offered to put Sandy and me up at a nearby hotel. Dr. H. thought a 2-block drive would be easier to handle than a 100-mile round trip drive. I was very grateful for Rob's generosity.

Friday October 22, 2004

Rachel and Val came by to visit. Rachel brought an earth toned ceramic chicken. She lived in an apartment with her sister and two other students. They shared the household chores. Whenever anyone ignored their chore, such as the dishes, one of them would place the chicken by the sink as a reminder that it was important to do the dishes. She set the chicken by my bed as a symbol that my care was important. The chicken became known as my cancer chicken. As a note, after Tom's diagnoses, I kept the chicken near him to signify the importance of his care. I still have the chicken.

Saturday, October 23, 2004

I would be discharged on Sunday and check into a near by hotel. Tom rented a wheelchair for me so I could get around the hotel suites. By this time, I was so weak I could hardly walk as far as the bathroom. I was grateful he thought to get one for me.

Sunday, October 24, 2004

The hotel suites gave us a medical discount of which I thought was very nice. I would be there until Thursday so it would be a long stay.

It was strange to walk into the hotel since Tom and I had stayed there a few years before. We had received a weekend gift. The main theme of this hotel was all the water, waterfalls, and the live ducks swimming around. What a wonderful and serene atmosphere to be in while I completed treatment.

The Dilaudid I was now on was very helpful. Combined with a morphine patch and a motion sickness patch, the combination made a dramatic difference for me. It controlled my pain to the point that it was tolerable. With the nausea under control and the pain under control and I felt much better.

Tom and Phillip bought some groceries for us for our stay at the hotel. They picked up some sandwiches for our dinner. My sister Lindalee brought some things as well, such as little comforts, like soft throws and fluffy pillows. After the room was set up, everyone left for the night. My appetite had improved, and I was able to eat part of the sandwich Tom had brought. Sandy ran the tub so I could have my evening soak, as I lay on the couch with my feet elevated. My feet were still swelling, and elevation did seem to relive them.

I asked Tom to stay home for a few days so he could save his energy and time to help me out once I got home. Tom left our small car for Sandy to use to drive the three blocks to the hospital for radiation treatment. Even though Sandy was nervous about driving, something she avoided, she felt confident she could handle three simple blocks.

Monday, October 26, 2004

My radiation treatment was schedule for the same time I had kept since the beginning. The hotel had free breakfast which including eggs and bacon. I have a weakness for bacon and found it surprisingly delicious that morning. We made lunch in our suite which had a stove, refrigeration, and micro-wave. Dishes were included, making it handy for a few days stay.

Sandy pushed me around the hotel in the wheelchair. Everyone working there knew I was a cancer patient. They were all helpful and nice to us. There were snacks at happy hour, but we did not go. It was nice at the hotel with Sandy's help. I got my four soaks a day, plenty of water and food whenever I felt like eating. Sandy still made sure I was drinking my nutritional drinks, so I had some intake.

Staying close to the hospital proved to be yet another key to my nausea. With such a short drive to the hospital, I did not experience all the discomforts physically as the long drive had caused.

Tuesday, October 27, 2004

I was still having difficulty with swollen legs and feet and found myself elevating my legs more often. My pain control was good which helped with my comfort and tolerance. Peeing still burned terribly but it was tolerable with the pain medication.

There was work going on down the block from the hotel.

They informed us that there would be some electricity interruptions but limited to a three-hour duration. Unfortunately, the three-hour interruption became six hours and after dark. The hotel gave us glow sticks to light the room. Sandy was still able to run my bath. The glow sticks gave the bathroom a soft glow as if candles surrounded me.

Wednesday, October 27, 2006

I was getting anxious for my radiation treatments to be come to an end. It had already been over seven weeks and I really wanted them done. I was so raw both front and back that I was not sure how much more I could stand. I was glad I was done with chemotherapy though. Both of them together were very rough to handle.

While Sandy and I were down by the ducks, I had a craving for a Pepsi, but all the machines sold were Coke. One of the workers was going by, so we asked if there was a machine that sold Pepsi. She said they had Pepsi in the employee's lounge and she would get me one.

When she brought it back to us, she refused to let us pay for it. I do not know why, but it tasted so good. To this day, it has become one of my comfort foods. It is funny how things come about, because, before that, I was not much of a pop drinker.

Sandy was becoming worn out from pushing me around in the wheelchair so when we got close to the room; I held onto the chair and walked about twenty feet. I wanted some exercise, but I did get exhausted so easily, but it was good to walk.

Thursday, October 28, 2004

I woke up very excited because I knew today was my last day of radiation therapy. I had been so upset over the last three days of treatment, because I had my heart set on Monday being the last day. That made the "new" last three days even harder. Val and Rob came and helped pack up our things. Val and I were going to drive home in our car and Sandy would ride with Rob. We went to treatment and then home. It felt so good to be home. I got comfortable on the couch and spent the rest of the day there. I was anxious to see Tom when he got home from work.

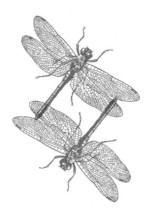

CHAPTER 6 - RITA'S RECOVERY

Friday, Saturday, Sunday Monday

October 29 – November 1, 2004

I do not remember much about these days. I know Sandy had me on a rigid schedule for eating, drinking and tub soaks. She did the laundry, cooking and house cleaning. Tom still sanitized the tub for my evening soak and sat in the bathroom with me. It was our quite time together. I do not remember watching the Packer game, but I am sure we did, but of course it could have been a bye week, but I don't remember.

Tuesday, November 2, 2004

Sandy took me to the town hall so I could vote. It is amazing the things we feel are important even when we are ill. Tom's brother, Dave, came for a visit. I am not sure the exact day, but it was nice of him to visit.

Thursday, November 4, 2004

My appointment with Dr. H. went well today. While we were waiting to see him, Sandy found me a Pepsi. It tasted good. Dr. H. said I was progressing very well and that my skin was looking good with no signs of infection. That was good news.

He also told me he was pleased that I had survived such an aggressive treatment. So was everyone else.

When you are going through cancer treatments, it hard to see the final outcome of those treatments. For me, it wasn't until I was actually done with treatment and began feeling better, that I realized how much I had been through. The results will be that I am cancer free, and that Tom and I can continue our lives together. My children will still have their mom and my parents will still have their daughter.

There were times during treatment that I really wanted to give up. My support group and my doctors just would not let that happen, good for them and good for me.

Friday, November 5, 2004

Since Sandy would be leaving for home tomorrow, Val and Rob wanted to take us all out for dinner. Val's daughter, Christina and her daughter, Heidi also came. The food looked and smelled so good, but I could not eat. I was in so much pain and extremely uncomfortable that all I wanted to do was go home. I knew Sandy would not have gone out if I had not come along and I wanted her to have a nice, fancy dinner. I just sat there and enjoyed everyone's company. I really wished I had an appetite because everything looked and smelled so good.

Saturday, November 6, 2004

Sandy left today. Tom and I took her to the airport. I was reluctant to let her go. She was so much help and support. Tom established a new relationship with her and had a lot of appreciation for all she had done for us. It was hard to see her go.

I continued my daily bath soaks and made sure I was drinking water. It was still hard to eat much but I drank my nutritional drinks "like a good little girl" as Sandy had said.

Monday, November 8, 2004

Kathy took me for my appointment with Dr. B. He said I was healing very well and that he could no longer felt any remains of the tumor. That was reassuring. I was scheduled for an anal ultra-sound for December 27, 2004. It was the soonest I could go since the radiation would continue to work for another four weeks, even though treatments were done.

I was still having leg and feet swelling. Dr B. explained that my lymph nodes in the groin area were destroyed by the radiation and the swelling was a result of that. The blood and fluids were not being returned throughout my body correctly.

I continued leg elevation to help reduce the symptoms and he would do a follow up on my next visit.

Tuesday, November 9, 2004

As I thought about all I had been through the past two months, I was astonished at where all the time had gone.

My eyes are blurring, and I cannot seem to focus, making writing very difficult. It had been a rough two months. It was truly the hardest thing I have ever done in my life. It was scary, painful, depressing and a major challenge. Now I need to wait until the anal ultra-sound to find out if treatments accomplished what they were supposed to do, to see if my cancer was gone.

Wednesday, November 10, 2004

Today is the best I have felt in months. My vision is still blurry. I have wanted to make some beaded jewelry, but my hands are shaky and since my eyes are blurry, I cannot see the beads to string them. Maybe I want too much too soon.

Trying to remember everything that has happened is difficult. Except for the things I actually wrote in my journal, the rest is from memory that I needed to verify with others who were there. I am happy that I am done with treatments.

I am still sleeping on the couch. My skin is still very tender, and I feel protective of it, so I am comfortable sleeping alone. I like the couch because I can use the back and pillows to get myself into the most comfortable position for sleeping.

Thursday – Thursday, November 11-16, 2004

I did not journal too much during this time. I am not sure why. I remember that Tom came home every day to make sure I had lunch. I only soaked in the tub two times per day. Early morning before Tom left for work and then again when he got home.

I am having difficulties walking. My legs would give out after about eight to ten feet. I still have the wheelchair and do use it to get around. I feel extremely fatigued. The nausea is getting better, but I still take the Compazine daily to keep it in check. My appetite is a little better, but I am still not interested in eating. I still like to drink Pepsi.

Wednesday, November 17, 2004

Today is Phillip's 24th birthday. I have always made a cake on someone's birthday and I did not want today to be any different. I got everything I needed to make the cake and put it on the counter. Then I sat and rested. I put it all into a bowl and then rested. I mixed up the ingredients and then rested. Put the ingredients in the pans, rested. Put them into the oven and rested. I did this until the cake was done. It must have taken me two hours before the whole cake was completed with decorations and all. Nevertheless, I felt good about being able to remember Phillip's birthday this way.

Friday, November 19, 2004

Gloria from Afton came to visit today. It was good to see her. Her cancer is gone, and she is making good progress on her recovery. She was back to work part-time and feels fatigued quite a bit. She is still taking heavy doses of pain medication and is hoping to be able to get off them soon. She explained that it has been very difficult for her to wean off them but is still trying.

It was encouraging for me to see her. It gave me hope that my cancer too, could be gone when I went for my ultra-sound in December. Then we both could be success stories.

Thursday, November 25, 2004

Tom and Phillip made a wonderful Thanksgiving dinner. Rachel and Valerie also helped. Everyone from my side of the family came. It was the most wonderful Thanksgivings that I can remember. I was very tired and could not help, but it was very nice to have everyone over to help celebrate my survival.

Friday, December 3, 2004

I drove today for the first time in months. It was a weird sensation. It required so much of my attention to be able to concentrate on what I was doing. I was still a little dizzy while driving, which surprised me because I did not seem so dizzy with just walking. I think the concentration required to drive well was a little more than I thought it would be. I took it slow and did not go too far.

Saturday, December 4, 2004

I decided to take off the motion sickness patch on Saturday and I became so sick. I was throwing up, nauseous, headache and dizziness. I even experienced hallucinations. It was bad. I put the patch back on and within a few hours, I felt like new. I am not sure how long I will need the patch, but as long as it works, I will use it. I think I have become addicted to it. I have an appointment with Dr. H. on Thursday of next week and we can discuss it then. I am still using the morphine patch as well and I know I am addicted to that.

Wednesday, December 8, 2004

I have finally gotten to the point where I do feel better. I am not where I want to be, but better than I was. I was beginning to think I would never get better. Impatient, I guess. I still experience fatigue and pain in my legs when I walk more than ten or fifteen feet. The swelling in my legs comes and goes. My skin is feeling much better. I only soak in the tub once day mostly because it is soothing. The skin damage seems to be healing, even though the skin is a deep, dark brown color.

Saturday, December 9, 2004

I met Gloria in Hudson today. It was good to see her. She is doing very well and looking much better. We ate lunch together and had a good visit. We plan to get together so we could meet each other's husbands and to celebrate our recoveries as soon as I get the "cancer free" diagnosis.

Saturday, December 11, 2004

Rachel and Valerie came over for a visit. They saw the wirework jewelry I had been working on. During my days after treatment, my vision remained unfocused. I missed working on my seed bead jewelry, but the seed beads were too small for my eyes to focus on and work with. My hands were a little unsteady as well.

I had some wire and large beads on hand, so I decided to try making wirework earrings using larger beads and some wire techniques. It worked out well and I had made over 20 pair of earrings over the past two weeks.

The girls saw the earrings I had made and asked if they could take them back to school with them. They were participating in an art sale the next week and thought my artistic earrings would fit in simply perfect. I agreed to let them have them.

After showing them to friends once they got home, they called and asked me if I could make some more before the sale began. I told them I would, and I could bring them over on Wednesday.

Wednesday, December 15, 2004

I managed to get several more pairs of earrings made as well as four wire and beaded necklaces done for the sale. I drove over to Menomonie and dropped them off with the girls. While I was there, we went out for lunch. It was nice spending quality time with them.

I took an Imodium before leaving them to assure myself I would make it all the way home. The driving was very tiring, and I was exhausted when I got home.

Thursday, December 16, 2004

I went to my appointment with Dr, H. by myself. It was in town, so it was not a long way to drive. He said my skin was healing quite well and beginning to look healthy again. We discussed the patches and my symptoms when I tried to take them off. He said we would address them at my next appointment and that I should not be concerned about getting off those medications right now.

I asked him about my lack of both bladder and bowel control. He told me he thought that there may be some permanent radiation damage to the two sphincter muscles, but we could determine the extent after my anal ultra-sound to verify that the cancer was gone.

I was content with that for now since my biggest concern

was the success of my cancer treatments.

Friday, December 17, 2004

I was surprised at how much energy I had today. I actually lasted long enough to get my and Tom's bedroom clean. I wanted to surprise him because I decided that I was ready to begin sleeping with him again. I no longer felt so protective on my skin and missed sleeping with Tom.

It would be nice to cuddle with him all night for the first time in months.

We both knew that making love was still out of the question for a while, but the idea of cuddling with him made me feel as though things had a chance of getting back to some degree of normalcy.

Saturday, December 18, 2004

We went to Tom's work Christmas party. I was very weak and tired, but I seemed important to me to be able to go. Everyone asked me how I was doing and was happy to see me active again. I did not eat too much because I wasn't very hungry, but I enjoyed the company. After dinner, Tom and I danced a slow dance together. Everyone clapped to share their happiness for us that I survived and were happy for both Tom and me. That was about as much evening out that I could handle, so we went home shortly thereafter. I was exhausted by the time we got home but did have a good evening.

Sunday, December 19, 2004

Today was a good day to watch football. I really enjoyed going out with Tom last night, but I feel tired from it. I was surprised that I did not get as tired as I usually had been getting. I feel encouraged that my physical health is returning.

Monday, December 20, 2004

The sale of my jewelry went well. Almost every piece sold. It feels good to have a sense of accomplishment after so many months of doing nothing but having treatments.

Friday, December 24, 2004

On Christmas Eve, we went to my sister Val and her boyfriend, Rob's house for dinner. I did not have a lot of energy, but it was enjoyable to see everyone. We stayed at a nearby hotel and left for home the next morning. **Saturday, December 25, 2004**

We spent Christmas day with just our daughters, Rachel and Valerie and their boyfriends and Phillip and his girlfriend. Tom and the children made dinner. It was nice to be a little low-keyed as I was feeling very tired from all the traveling.

Sunday, December 26, 2004

We went to Gordon to celebrate Christmas with Tom's side of the family.

My visit with his family was limited to me lying on the couch most of the time. I was so exhausted that I could do little else. It was fun to watch them share gifts, conversation, and humor. We went home that night, as I really wanted to sleep in my own bed.

Ultra-sound Day
Monday, December 27, 2004

I was very apprehensive as Tom, and I drove over to Minneapolis for my anal ultra-sound and the results of my cancer treatments. Tom was very quiet.

I changed my lower half into a gown and lay on my side on the exam table. Dr. F. talked softly as he conducted the test.

When he said that he could hardly tell that any tumor had ever been present at all, I began to cry from sheer joy.

After getting dressed, I was so anxious to tell Tom, I could hardly wait to get back to the waiting room.

I know Tom already knew the answer by the expression on my face, but I said it anyhow.

"I am cancer free!"

He held me tightly for a few minutes and I could tell he was greatly relieved that we could "grow old together".

New Year's Eve - January 2005

As was Tom's tradition each New Year's Eve, he cooked a lobster dinner. I always found it such a sweet and romantic time for us to bring in the New Year. This New Year was especially joyful because we could see a wonderful future ahead of us. I had survived cancer.

Monday, January 3, 2005

Tom took me for my appointment with Dr. B. He said I was doing quite well and that he was happy that my most recent test showed that I was negative for cancer. He said my skin was healing quite well and my overall health seemed greatly improved. It was so nice to hear those words. I had been through so much and realized it had all been worth the pain and worry. It made my heart joyous.

Tuesday, January 11, 2005

I have been feeling tired the past few days and have noticed that I am having problems with my breathing. My lungs hurt when I breathe, and I can't seem to get enough air.

Wednesday, January 12, 2005

I went to the clinic today regarding my breathing difficulties. My doctor put me on three different medications all to treat respiratory difficulties.

Thursday, January 13, 2005

I am still having difficulty with breathing. My chest feels tight, and it still hurts to take a breath. The medications I received do not seem to be helping. I am struggling more each day. I cannot sleep and I think I should go to the doctor again to find out what is happening. I am reluctant since I have spent so much time in hospitals and at doctors. I will wait a few more days to see it my breathing pain improves.

Third Hospitalization - Pneumonia

Saturday, January 15, 2005

Tom took me to the emergency room because I my breathing was so labored and I couldn't take any deep breathes, just little, painful puffs. I was admitted to the hospital with pneumonia. Poor Tom, he has been through enough and now this. I was surprised that I had pneumonia.

I found it difficult to breathe even after treatment began. I was anxious all the time and could not find the peace to sleep. The nurse played soft relaxation music for me but that did not help. I was so afraid of not being able to breathe that I could not relax.

Sunday, January 16, 2005

My doctor and I discussed and decided to remove the two patches. I could tell my anxiety level increased and the nightmares started again. After three days, I seemed less nauseous and hallucinogenic. I was relieved to know I was going to be able to get off the morphine. I have never been much of a drug user, so it did give me some peace of mind to know the need for it had passed. Tom and Phillip came to visit each day. Jessie, Phillip's girlfriend, came with Phillip one day as well. It was nice to see her support for Tom, Phillip, and me.

Wednesday, January 19, 2005

My red blood count dropped to 7.6 and I received a blood transfusion. I am once again beginning to worry if I was ever going to get better. My body had been through so many traumas I wondered how long it was going to take to improve. My legs continue to be weak while the pain in my hips does not seem to be improving. I felt confident that I was on my way to recovery since the cancer tumor was now gone. The fear that it would return remained in my subconscious though.

Thursday, January 20, 2005

I noticed how much better I feel today. It is amazing how healthy blood can make you feel so much better. I forgot my sister Val's birthday yesterday, but I am sure she will forgive me.

I am very happy the cancer is gone. I was not sure what kind of trade-off there would be to obtain a cure for the cancer. I have been having tests all this week such as blood, heart tests and x-rays. As of now, its high blood pressure, diabetes, damaged lymph nodes, damaged bladder, and damaged sphincter muscle and a heart murmur. I do remember reading somewhere that chemotherapy could result in some heart damage.

I have a lot to digest. I must consider my future ambitions, occupation, house chores, finances and values. In addition, my health and all these conditions I now must deal with. I am not certain if any of them are permanent or if they will improve with time.

I am angry. I did ok accepting that I had cancer, but why all this new stuff? Wasn't it enough to go through all of it and endure the healing? I do not understand why all the added baggage. I feel that my family has already endured enough. I cannot help but wonder why my family and I have to endure even more.

I am confused. I have so much health and personal issues to deal with that I do not know where to begin. I feel like a wreck. Maybe this is what all cancer survivors go through. I am not sure, but I know I want some peace from all of it, even for just a little while.

Friday, January 21, 2005

I had to call school and cancel my Native American presentation for the fifth-grade classes. I looked forward to that each year, but I do not know if I will be out of the hospital in time to give it or even be able to physically handle it.

Saturday, January 22, 2005

I was released from the hospital today. I was sent home with so much medical stuff and instructions, which I was glad that Tom understood what I was supposed to do and take. I had a nebulizer with two types of medications. Some antibiotics and a blood sugar monitor device. I could not understand how I suddenly developed Type 2 diabetes. I was determined to have that re-checked in the near future. (Note: the Type 2 diabetes showed up from the blood in the transfusion. Later discover I did not have it.)

My personal doctor put me on an anti-anxiety medication and heart medications as well. I continue to take the anti-depressant I was started on in October.

For now, I am determined to stay on top of any symptoms or changes in my body that may need immediate attention. I am hopeful that many of the new conditions are temporary and will take care of themselves as my body heals and my health returns.

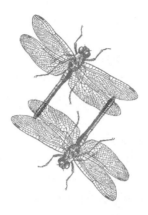

CHAPTER 7 - TOM'S DIAGNOSIS AND TREATMENTS

Monday, January 24, 2005

Tom has been coughing a lot lately and having problems with his breathing. I am wondering if it is the same cough from last September. Maybe he got my pneumonia. Either way I asked him to go to the doctor, no excuses. He told me he would make an appointment for this week.

Friday, January 28, 2005

After four more days of coughing, Tom finally went to the doctor.

After x-rays were completed, Tom was diagnosed with pneumonia with a suspicious left hilar mass. The hilar is related to the hilum of the lung structure. This is where the root of the lung is located, and air enters and leaves the lungs. Blockage of this area is causing Tom's breathing difficulties. His doctor put him on oral antibiotics of 500 mg daily of Levaquin. He also prescribed an Albuterol inhaler to use 4-6 times daily.

Wednesday, February 2, 2005

Tom went to the doctor again today. He is not improving.

This time his doctor did a CT. We should have the results in a few days. In the meantime, his doctor put him on an IV antibiotic. Tom is receiving the IV treatment in the chemotherapy department.

Thursday, February 3, 2005

I went with Tom for his second IV treatment. He is still feeling a little drowsy, so I drove. His breathing has not improved.

Friday, February 4, 2005

Tom went to work today. During his lunch, he went for his third IV treatment. We have not heard from the doctor about the results of his February 2nd CT.

Saturday, February 5, 2005

Tom had his fourth IV treatment today. He does not seem to be getting better with this treatment. Even with the IV antibiotics, Tom is not improving. I am concerned about his health at this point. I am trying to put my health issues on the back burner so I can concentrate on Tom's issues.

Sunday, February 6, 2005

Tom and I went for his fifth IV treatment. No one was in the chemotherapy department, so a second-floor nurse took care of it for him.

Monday, February 7, 2005

I called Tom's doctor for the results of his CT, but he refused to give them to me. He said he could only give the results to Tom and wanted Tom to come in tomorrow so they could discuss it.

In the meantime, I got some more tests result back. My diabetic test came back "normal". It appears that my personal doctor was jumping the gun again with yet another wrong diagnosis. My count for the diabetic test was five, which is normal. We spent all that money for diabetic supplies we did not need in the first place, of which the insurance would not pay for.

In addition, my most recent heart test came back normal after my doctor panicked in the hospital saying it was dangerously abnormal. My blood pressure was 98/60 so she decided to have me stop one of the two blood pressure medications she had put me on while I was in the hospital. I have lost my faith in her. I made up my mind that I will consider a different doctor at the clinic for my personal doctor. She has made to many mistakes for me to take the chance with my future health to keep her as my doctor.

The best news I received was that my red blood count was 11.08. Fantastic! I think getting off the patches and discontinuing the Dilaudid helped my body to start a natural balance.

Tom's Lung Cancer
Tuesday, February 8, 2005

Tom, and I went to the appointment today to learn the results of his recent CT test. It was not a good appointment as if was full of bad news. His doctor said he suspected that Tom might have lung cancer. What? Did I understand this? Cancer? Haven't we had enough? How could that be? I am hoping that is a big mistake.

His doctor explained that the CT indicated a large lobulated (consisting of many lobes) mass sitting in the middle of both lungs. The mass was located in the middle mediastinum and on the left upper and lower lobes. Also involved is the hilar component engulfing the left main stem bronchus. As the doctor was describing the radiology findings, I began to fear that his suspicion of cancer was possible.

To rule out cancer, Tom needed to have a lung biopsy done. He further explained that Dr. M. at a hospital in St. Paul would do the biopsy. He also added that there was an Adrenal mass, of which we could address after the lung biopsy.

I could feel my world crashing down around me. I hoped with all my heart that it was not cancer. I have not even recovered yet, how could we handle more.

Shortly after we got home, we received a phone call to set up Tom's Bronchoscopy and lung biopsy for the next day. That was quick.

Tom and I did not discuss the possibility of him having

cancer. Maybe if we did not talk about it, it would not be true. How could it be? We were both full of fear that once again, those three little words, "You have cancer" would once again invade into our lives.

Lung biopsy Procedure Thoracoscopy
Thursday, February 10, 2005

There are four procedures used to obtain a lung biopsy, they are: Bronchoscope, needle, open or video-assisted thorascopic surgery (VATS). VATS uses a scope, which passes through a small chest incision to remove a sample of tissue.

Phillip and I took Tom to a hospital in St. Paul for his lung biopsy. Lindalee and Jeff met us there. It was good to have their support.

The doctor used Fiberoptic Bronchoscope method for Tom's biopsy. This method passes a small tube through his nose and down into the lungs. The biopsy will be taken through this scope.

Tom was sedated and we were asked to leave. I felt helpless as I left his room. I was full of fear because in my heart I knew it was cancer. I tried to get that thought out of my mind, but it would not go away.

The procedure took about 45 minutes and Tom went to recovery. The doctor came to the waiting area to speak with us. He confirmed our fears. It was cancer. He said it was small cell neuroendocrine carcinoma and was sitting in the middle of both lungs but more concentrated on the lower left lobe. He told us it was inoperable. My heart just broke. Even though, I was full of hope. I beat my cancer and now Tom needed to beat his.

We went to the recovery room to see Tom. He was quite groggy but awake. He said his throat hurt. Then he wanted to know what the doctor found out. I told him and I could see the dismay in his face.

At this point, he just wanted to go home. He has such a strong disposition that the nurse had to talk him into staying a little longer. Sometimes he is so stubborn. After his release, he was anxious to go.

The doctor instructed us to contact Tom's doctor to set up a CT to see if the cancer had metastasized anywhere else. When we got home, I called to set up a CT for Tom. To my surprise, it was scheduled for the next day.

Friday, February 11, 2005

When we arrived at the radiation department at our local hospital for Tom's CT an eerie feeling crept over me. We had been there so many times for me but now it was for Tom.

Tom had a CT with contrast. The purpose of the CT was to determine if the cancer had moved to the lymph nodes, brain, abdomen or the bones. Since we were not yet seeing an oncologist, I suspected it would be a few days until we got the results. When I was seeing Dr. H., he got the test results almost immediately.

Tom's doctor completed a referral for Tom to see Dr. H. This gave me hope. I have a strong trust in Dr. H. and his skills as an oncologist and a doctor.

Saturday February 12, 2005

Tom and I went to the casino for a night out. He does enjoy going there. On the way to the casino, I tried to talk to him about the cancer, but he did not have much to say.

"I can beat it, you know", he told me, "Just like you beat yours. Remember, we are supposed to grow old together."

Tuesday, February 14, 2005

This Valentine's Day was not a happy one. The past week has been a living hell and was getting worse as the days went by.

We got Tom's results back. He not only had small cell lung cancer, but the cancer had metastasized to his brain where they found multiple tumors and also tumors in his adrenal glands.

I am angry. It is not fair for us to have to endure so much hardship in so little time. Why us? Why now? Before my diagnosis of cancer, the past two years had been some of the happiest years Tom and I have spent together.

We were falling back in love and were enjoying our time together. We had made some wonderful plans and talked about our dreams. If he dies, that is all gone. I want to spend many, many years with him. After all, that is what got me through my cancer, so we could grow old together? I feel like I am going to go crazy. I do not know if I can handle this.

Tom has an appointment with Dr. H. on Thursday.

We decided not to tell our family about the cancer until we knew more. We thought after Tom's appointment with Dr. H. would be the best.

Thursday, February 17, 2005

Today was one of the most devastating and heart-breaking days I have ever experienced in my life. We went to see Dr. H. He seemed reluctant to give us the news about Tom's cancer. I had gotten to know Dr. H. well over the past five months of my treatment and he had gotten to know Tom and me. I could tell it was hard for him to give us the news. I never expected what he was about to say.

He said, "I really hate to tell you this, but your cancer is terminal." My eyes began to burn with tears and my heart became so heavy in my chest it was crushing me.

Tom said, "What do you mean? Am I going to die?"

Dr. H. paused, "I am sorry to have to say this. You have extensive stage lung cancer, and it is quite advanced with brain metastases. You have about nine months, maybe twelve. I am so sorry."

He quietly left the room so Tom and I could be alone.

The tears were falling from both of our eyes. Our hearts were breaking. We just held each other and cried. We had no words for each other. What could we say?

A short while later Dr. H. returned. He explained that Tom not only had lung cancer but also metastases to his brain and adrenals. Tom's cancer was small cell neuroendocrine carcinoma. He explained the drug and treatments Tom would receive which included whole brain radiation. Dr. H. wanted to start chemotherapy within a few days of the start of Tom's radiation treatments. The Chemotherapy drugs Dr. H. was going to use were Cisplatin and Etoposide.

Tom asked, "Will I get as sick as Rita did?"

Dr. H. replied, "No, Rita had an extremely aggressive treatment program. She went to hell and back. I'm not taking you that far."

He told us that Dr. B. would be Tom's radiologist. I felt comfortable with that decision and confident in Tom's future treatments because I already knew all the people who would be involved with his care. After all, they were the same people who had taken care of me.

Dr. H. also suggested that Tom make a Living Will and a Financial Will. He then suggested that Tom apply for Social Security Disability and meet with the Social Worker.

Tom received a prescription for dexamethasone, which is a steroid to prevent edema. Edema is the accumulation of fluids beneath the skin. In Tom's case it was for his brain. He would be undergoing full brain radiation. He will continue with his Lisinopril and Verapamil to control his high blood pressure of which he has had for several years.

It was a quiet ride home. Tom did not want to talk about what the doctor had told us. I did not either. To say it aloud would only make it real. I was so angry at life at that moment. I was dreading the task we had once we got home.

We had to tell his family and then mine. What a difficult thing to do. It was only five months earlier that we were telling them about my cancer. I felt this whole thing was unfair and how cruel for us to have to do this again. We saved telling the girls until last. Phillip already knew Tom had cancer, but he did not know it was terminal.

The reaction to the news was the same total disbelief that this awful thing was happening to us again.

Within a few hours of telling the girls, they arrived at our door. Once again, they were armed with nutritional ideas and supplements especially designed for lung cancer.

These supplements included amino acids in the form of Cysteine and carotenoids such as Lycopene, which inhibits the proliferation of cancer cells involved in lung cancer. Foods they encouraged were bee pollen, which increase the life span of lung cancer patients and a variety of fruits due to their Phenethyl Isothiocyanate content, such as grapes, raspberries, and strawberries. Phenethyl Isothiocyanate help to kill the cancer cells implicated in lung and other types of cancers.

Before adding any supplements to your diet during cancer treatments, talk it over with your doctor. Some supplements or foods can cause toxicity or interfere with certain chemotherapy drugs.

I know the girls spent many hours doing this research and I cannot even imagine what thoughts were going through their heads when they heard they had a second parent with cancer.

Brian Radiation
Friday, February 18, 2005

Tom and I went to his appointment in St. Paul with Dr. B. It was strange to be back again, only this time for Tom's treatments. The therapists offered their sincere support for us and assured us that they would take good care of Tom. I knew they would since they had taken such good care of me.

Tom went through many of the same procedures that I had; except he was fitted with a mesh face/head mold called an Aquaplast mask. The mask is made from a thermoplastic mesh, wetted, and easily fitted to the facial structure of each individual patient. Once this mask dries, it becomes hardened. The edges are locked into place on the treatment table. This is placed on Tom's face each time he has radiation to keep him from moving and to keep the radiation field the same with each treatment.

Tom told Dr. B. he wanted to start treatment today, so Tom had his first whole-brain radiation treatment. I cringed as I watched the therapists lock the mesh mold down onto Tom's face and secure his head to the table. I cringed as the radiation machine began. I remember being in the same spot. It was the same therapists, the same room, and the same machine.

Metastasized Small Cell Neuroendocrine Carcinoma - Lung

Saturday, February 19, 2005

I did research on Tom's type of cancer. A neuroendocrine tumor originates in relationship with endocrine (hormonal) system and nervous system. The endocrine system communicates with the hormones and acts as a messenger to regulate the production and secretion of hormones. It is an important but complicated system but is directly related to Tom's type of cancer.

The lungs are an uncommon site for this type of cancer to spread. Most neuroendocrine tumors are slow growing, with the exception of small cell neuroendocrine carcinoma, which is highly malignant, fast growing. It is rare. Unfortunately, this is the type that Tom has.

It feels ironic that my cancer is rare and so is Tom's cancer.

As I did research on the lungs, I did not realize how complex they are. The chest cavity where the lungs are located includes a space called the mediastinum. The mediastinum is the center of the chest and contains the lymph nodes, thymus and the heart. The mediastinum separates the left and right lung from each other. If the chest wall is punctured on the left side, causing the left lung to collapse, the fight lung remains inflated and functioning, because of the separation by the mediastinum.

One of the locations of Tom's cancer is the middle mediastinum. I can now comprehend why Tom's cancer is inoperable. Added to the complication of the cancer location in the lungs is the metastasis to the brain.

Tom's brain tumors were located in various locations in the cerebellum. The cerebellum has two-cerebellar hemispheres one left and one right. Each hemisphere controls that side of the body's functions, left controls left and right controls right. Several tumors were located in the right cerebellar hemisphere, the right frontal lobe and the right temporal lobe. The largest one was located in the left parietal lobe. There were others scattered throughout as well. The tumors had metastases to numerous sections of Tom's brain.

Again, the brain is more complicated than I realized, but

from the report, I knew that the locations of the tumors would eventually interfere with his functions in the future.

Monday, February 21, 2005

Tom had his second radiation treatment today. He drove. Tom's radiation treatments are in the late afternoon, so he works until lunch and then we drive to St. Paul.

As I watched Tom receive his treatment, I remembered how destructive and damaging radiation was to my tissues. Now they were using this horrible process on Tom's brain. I began to cry and tried to hide my tears.

One of the therapists gave me a hug and said they would do their best for Tom. I knew they would, but at that moment, that gave me no comfort.

After his radiation treatment, Tom and I went to the cancer center for the Chemotherapy Class. We received some handouts and a curriculum to follow. There were about twenty people in the class. It consisted of cancer patients and their care-givers. I was the only survivor present as a caregiver.

I would like to think that my presence there as a cancer survivor, especially one who had chemotherapy, offered some hope to the others present.

The curriculum covered why and how chemotherapy is used. The possible side effects of treatment were discussed as well as how to deal with those side effects.

Tuesday, February 22, 2005

After Tom's third radiation, we went to the second session of the chemotherapy classes in the cancer center. Subjects we learned about were understanding chemotherapy, side effects, fatigue, and symptoms to report to the nurse. Written information we received were brochures and booklets relating to chemotherapy and support group meetings.

So far, Tom feels good but is apprehensive about starting chemotherapy tomorrow. I am apprehensive as well.

I am still on my anti-depressant, which is probably a good thing at this point in my life. I am still in shock that Tom has cancer. It is hard to believe that our lives continue to evolve around radiation, chemotherapy and many hours spent in hospitals.

Cycle One - Chemotherapy
Wednesday, February 23, 2005

Tom had a slight headache and had difficulty sleeping last night.

After Tom's fourth radiation treatment, we went down to the cancer center, a place I am awfully familiar with, to start Tom's chemotherapy treatment. He began cycle one of session one. There would be four sessions in cycle one. Tom is receiving chemotherapy drugs called Cisplatin on day one and Cytoxan for days two and three. He will receive Etoposide each day of each session.

Tom got an IV line placed into his arm. We were provided with information about these drugs, but as I was reading all the possible side effects, I decided I really did not want to know. I read the information any way. Some of the possible side effects could or could not be permanent. They included possible kidney and nerve damage, hearing loss, hair loss and nausea and vomiting.

I assumed that hair loss would happen since a side effect of the Etoposide was also hair loss. Other side effects of the Etoposide are decreased white and red blood counts and the reduction of platelets. Lowered platelets cause concern for excessive bleeding and bruising. It could also cause mouth sores.

The nurse started the drug, Cisplatin. This took three hours to complete. When the Cisplatin finished, the nurse started the Topiside. This drug took an additional two hours to complete. To pass the time, we watched video movies for a while. Tom became sleepy from the anti-nausea medication Zofran, the same drug I had also received. He did sleep for a while. It was a very long day. Tom had a slight headache by the time we left the treatment. I drove home. Tom was sent home with a prescription of Zofran.

I was not sure if I felt exhausted because of the long day or

RITA K MILLER KASINSKAS

if my body was not ready for all the activity it was enduring. Either way, Tom and I took a nap for a few hours.

Thursday February 24, 2005 - Chemotherapy

Tom did not sleep well last night and still had his headache this morning.

We drove over to St Paul for Tom's fifth brain radiation treatment and went to the cancer center for his second session of his first cycle of chemotherapy.

Tom is taking the three days of his chemotherapy off from work. He seemed to be handling it quite well, but we spent all day in St. Paul, so there was no time left for him to go to work.

The day went much the same as it had yesterday, except Tom did not want the Zofran. He said it made him tired. He said he did not want to feel so tired. We watched video movies most of the afternoon. He was not hungry but drank some soda pop.

Friday February 25, 2005 – Chemotherapy

Tom went to his sixth brain radiation treatment and then back down for chemotherapy for session three of his first cycle. I was doing the driving because the treatments were beginning to exhaust him. We had lunch while we were there for treatment. Tom seems to be eating OK today. He was never much of a lunch eater, so when he did not want to eat, I was not worried. He did drink a lot of juice and water.

Sunday, February 27, 2005

Each year for Kathy's birthday we traditionally do something special for her. We had already planned to go to the casino for an overnight, but since Tom was in treatment, I told Tom I would not go. Tom said I should go. Phillip said he would keep Tom company and not to worry. I decided I would go since I felt I needed a time out from all the things that were going on in my life. Tom was not getting sick with his treatment like I had, so I decided it would be good for me to spend some time with Kathy.

Monday February 28, 2005

Phillip went with Tom for his seventh radiation treatment. After treatment, Tom went to work. He did not have chemotherapy today. His next cycle is not due until the second week of March.

I had a relaxing time with Kathy, but I got nauseous when I went into Jacuzzi. I enjoy swimming in the pool but only for a short while. The little trip did tire me out though. I worried about Tom while I was gone, but upon returning home, I realized that he was doing quite well.

Tuesday, March 1, 2005

Tom is feeling better this week. He had his eighth radiation treatment today. He told me that he is feeling fine and wanted to drive back and forth to treatments. He did mention that he seemed to be having a hard time hearing. I became worried about this, because one possible side effect of Cisplatin was hearing loss. Of course, the brain radiation may be affecting his hearing as well. I cleaned his ears with wax remover, and it seemed to help a little.

Wednesday, March 2, 2005

Tom had his ninth radiation treatment today. He told me that his is still having hearing problems but also, he has developed a ringing in his ears. I made note to have Tom ask Dr. H. about this at Tom's next appointment.

Thursday, March 3, 2005

After Tom's tenth radiation treatment, he went to work. I have noticed that Tom seems to be having some difficulty concentrating and he seems forgetful. When he got home, however, he did remember to call our brother-in-law, Larry and wish him a happy birthday.

Friday, March 4, 2005

Today I noticed that Tom is starting to lose some of his hair. It is just small amounts, but I am sure that once he has his next chemotherapy, it will all fall out. Tom has not mentioned how he feels at the prospect of losing his hair.

He had his eleventh radiation treatment today. I am anxious for these treatments to be done.

Saturday, March 5, 2005

Tom has decided to take it easy today. He had been pushing himself so hard during this last set of treatments, it is a wonder he can even function. He does not talk to me very much about this whole process, so I have decided to let him have his space. When he is ready to talk, I will listen.

Sunday, March 6, 2005

Tom's brother Marty and his wife, Lynnette came for a visit. Tom had not seen his brother since Christmas; it was good to see Tom and he have an enjoyable visit.

Monday, March 7, 2005

Tom had his eleventh radiation today and he continues to drive. I told him I did not mind driving, but he said he is feeling better, not as tired.

Tuesday, March 8, 2005

I went to the doctor today after Tom's radiation treatment. I have a bladder infection and I am taking an antibiotic. I am continuing to use an anxiety medication and an anti-depressant. I know I am pushing myself beyond my physical ability. I continue to have leg and hip pain and the repeated bladder infections only complicate my recovery.

Wednesday, March 9, 2005

I drove to Tom's thirteenth treatment today. He said he was feeling tired and did not feel like fighting the traffic. Once we got home, he spent some time on the internet.

Thursday, March 10, 2005

Tom and I both had an appointment with Dr. H. today. Our times were back-to-back, so we went into the exam room together. Dr. H. addressed my recuperation and any problems I was having. After that, he addressed any of Tom's concerns or questions.

Tom told him that he was experiencing some hearing problems and ringing in his ears. Dr. H. said he would set up an appointment with a hearing specialist for him.

Dr. H. reviewed the list of the supplements Tom was taking and he asked him to stop taking his selenium, niacin, apricot seeds, and garlic. He explained that his chemotherapy would be more affective without these supplements. Dr. H. continued Tom on the anti-seizure medications and added an antidepressant.

Tom then asked Dr. H. if he could have his chemotherapy in our local hospital, since he would be done with radiation treatments in the cities today. Dr. H. said he would make those arrangements.

After our appointments, we went to St. Paul for Tom's fourteenth and last brain radiation treatment. I was relieved that his radiation was done with for now. I cannot imagine the damage it has done to his brain tissues. I hate to think about it.

I did notice Tom is still having some difficulty with his short-term memory. I forgot to ask Dr. H. about it. I forgot my list of questions to ask Dr, H. We will have to discuss this at the next appointment.

FMLA (Family and Medical Leave Act)
Friday, March 11, 2005

Tom applied for FMLA (Family and Medical Leave Act), to help protect his employment. His employer met the criteria of having 50 or more employees and Tom met the criteria of having worked at least 1,250 hours over the past 12 months.

He can miss twelve weeks of work. It is accumulative, meaning that if he misses one day this week and two days a few weeks later, it is only three days in the three-week period. His group health benefits are also protected by FMLA. I hope that it will be enough to get him through the year. He does talk about these issues. I know Tom's health benefits are very important right now and it does concern him.

Tuesday, March 15, 2005

It was nice that Tom had a break from treatments this week. His energy seems to be coming back and he is less tired. He feels better about work and it has been good for him to be able to put in his regular hours. Tomorrow he starts Chemotherapy again.

Cycle Two – Chemotherapy
Wednesday March 16, 2005

Tom started cycle two, session one of his chemotherapy at our local hospital. It was much easier to drive six miles rather than fifty miles. This is the first session of cycle two. He will miss three days of work this week since the chemotherapy is once again an all-day event. Tom did not want the Zofran again, but he was complaining that he was a little nauseous.

Thursday, March 17, 2005 - Chemotherapy

Tom has his second session of cycle two of chemotherapy today. His hair is starting to fall out. He told me that he wanted me to shave his head. He did not want hair falling out all over everything as he moved around. I shaved his head as close as I could get it. I kept a lock of his hair, for me.

I totally forgot to ware green today. Hope my mom does not find out. We have always had so much fun on St. Patrick's Day.

Friday March 18, 2005 - Chemotherapy

I am trying to remember my state of mind when I was going through treatment so I can empathize with Tom as he goes through his. Today he had his third session of cycle one of chemotherapy. I have noticed that he is very irritable lately.

I cannot be angry or blame him when he is over demanding because it hurts to have treatment. It messes up your mind and body. What he does not realize is that I am still in recovery. I try to make up for him and his chores, like the trash and other things, but I still get very tired.

I not only feel obligated to Tom because of love, but also because he stood by me throughout my treatments. It is difficult to be the female of a cancer couple. When I was going through treatment, my sister Sandy took a month off from her job and came here to help us. She flew from Oregon, leaving her husband, Larry, at home alone. Her husband has many medical problems himself. I know it was a difficult decision for them to make.

Sandy not only tended to my needs, but all the household chores such as laundry, cleaning, and cooking. This freed Tom up so he would miss as little work as possible. Little did I know how important that would become in our future lives.

During and after my treatment, my outside appearance was such that I looked cured and healed. Of course, no one could understand how devastating fatigue can be. I could barely walk 20 feet without becoming weak and tired.

Since I appeared better, the outside world assumed, including Tom, that I could just swing right back into things. Tom does not understand. How could he? He had never been there. Now that he is, it does not register because he is so consumed with trying to survive.

I have been dealing with a headache and irritability for over a week. I think because I am not where I want to be health wise has something to do with it. Carrying a laundry basket down the stairs and back up again is almost exhausting. I do not feel a sense of ambition at all. I almost feel lazy. However, each time I try to get things done, I feel so very tired. I though by now I would have a higher level of energy.

I know my worry about Tom's health is not helping matters. I still cannot believe we are once again dealing with cancer.

Sunday March 20, 2005

It is the first day of spring and is about 40 degrees outside. We have four inches of snow yesterday, but today the sun is helping to melt it. I seem to have more energy, but I still get tired easily. Tom is still having problems with his hearing, but his appetite seems good.

Monday, March 21, 2005

I am very excited about Wednesday. It is Tom's birthday and Sandy and her husband, Larry, have a wonderful surprise for him. They are flying in from Oregon on the twenty-third without Tom knowing, to celebrate his birthday with him. It is so hard to keep this secret. I cannot tell anyone to make sure it does not accidently slip out.

Tom has not seen Larry in a long time.

Tuesday, March 22, 2005

Tomorrow is Tom's 51st birthday. He is very tired but makes it to work every day. His hearing loss is very frustrating to him. I have been de-waxing his ears every day, but it only helps a little and only in one ear.

Tom's doctor put him on Cipro HC Otic, an antibiotic for the outer ear, to use in each ear four times a day. He is also on an oral antibiotic. Tom has an appointment with an ear specialist on March 31, 2005.

I hope the visit from Sandy and Larry lifts Tom's spirits.

Wednesday, March 23, 2005

I did the usual decorating with balloons, streamers, and signs for Tom. It's funny how he still loves the attention and hoop-la at his age. All three of our children were home for the evening surprise that none knew was going to happen.

Sandy and Larry made it to the cities just fine. They went to see Larry's mother Dora, first, since it is her birthday too. After visiting with Dora, they drove over to our house. Sandy was on her cell phone talking to Tom wishing him a happy birthday as they approached the end of our driveway. Tom had no idea. She continued to talk to Tom on her phone as she walked in the door.

Tom was so overwhelmed with surprise and happiness that he began to cry. What a wonderful surprise!

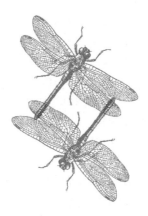

CAPTER 8 - CHANGES WITHIN EVERYDAY LIFE

In some cultures, the dragonfly, being a creature of the wind, represents change. One thing that remains constant, as one journeys through cancer, is change. It seems like everything in your life changes. There are a lot of adjustments to make and many new things to consider.

As I have mentioned, cancer takes the marriage vows of "In Sickness and In Health" to new depths. Love between a couple dealing with cancer needs to be strong and enduring. Two dragonflies together represent love. Tom and I are like the two dragonflies, holding onto our love as we deal with all the changes we are experiencing.

As Tom and I continue our journey through cancer, we are adjusting daily to change and cling daily to our love to survive. Everyday life becomes new and different.

As Tom and I journey along, everyday life must still be maintained and dealt with. Not just our lives but also those of our families and journeys they are on as well.

Thursday March 24, 2005

Tom, Sandy, and Larry all have their birthdays in March. To celebrate, we booked two rooms at the local casino. Mom and

Dad stayed in one room while Tom, I, Sandy, and Larry stayed in another room. We had a very nice dinner and decided to play some machines. Sandy and I were together when we heard our names paged. The page told us to go to security office. We looked at each other and the first thought we had was that something had happened to Tom.

When we got to the office, there was our mom on a gurney. She was experiencing a heart attack and the ambulance was on its way. Dad rode in the ambulance while Sandy and I followed in our car. Tom and Larry went back to the hotel as Tom was feeling tired.

The ER doctor said he felt it might be an artery in her heart. He explained that he would conduct some tests and we would know more in the morning. Since she was stable, the doctor told us to go back to the hotel and they would take good care of her. It was already getting late, so we took his advice.

Friday, March 25, 2005

We woke to a freezing hotel room. The heat had gone out during the night making the room very cold. No sooner then we realized the heat was out; there was a knock on the door. To my surprise, it was my dad. He explained that the doctor had mom transported to the Duluth hospital for emergency surgery.

The artery in her heart needed to immediate repair. She was already on her way, and dad was anxious to get to Duluth as soon as possible. He left right away.

While my dad was traveling to Duluth, mom had her surgery, placing a stent into her into her artery. Sandy and Larry went to Duluth to give support to my dad.

Tom was so worn out and tired, we went home.

Sandy and Larry decided to stay in Gordon with dad to drive him back and forth to Duluth while mom was in the hospital. Mom was doing well, but the doctor said he was not certain when she could go home. Since Sunday would be Easter and neither mom nor dad could make it to Tom's birthday/Easter dinner, Sandy and Larry decided to stay in Gordon.

I felt badly that they could not make it for Tom's party

because in my heart I feared it might be his last. I hoped it would not be, but the possible did exist.

Saturday, March 26, 2005

Mon is still in the hospital but is doing well. She might be able to go home today and spend Easter at her own house.

Sunday March 27, 2005

Sandy and Larry were still in Duluth with my parents. I really missed them today. Lindalee, Jeff, Tom's mother, Mary, and his brothers Marty and Al, came over for Tom's birthday and Easter dinner.

Once again, our children were instrumental in helping to get the dinner ready for all our guests. I wished more of Tom's family could have been here. Again, I am afraid it might be Tom's last birthday.

With Tom's hair completely gone, including his eyelashes and eyebrows, the Easter pictures were the first ones of him with his hair gone. He said it did not bother him emotionally. His only complaint was that the pillow irritated his head. I bought him a satin pillow cover and he said that made a difference.

Monday March 28, 2005

My emotions are very confusing these days. Even though I am on anti-depressants, my emotions are hard to figure out. Most of the time I feel "level", not depressed but not excited either. The past few days have been a real test of my feelings.

After mom had her heart attack, I was not as upset as I think I once would have been. I was concerned and worried for her, but not panicky. Maybe I am numb from all the things going on in our lives.

Thursday March 31, 2005

Sandy and Larry went home today. It was a weird visit with them spending a lot of time in Duluth. After mom got home from the hospital, it was already time for them to go home.

We found out today at Tom's hearing appointment that he has a significant hearing loss, and the doctor seems to believe that the Cisplatin chemotherapy drug is causing the loss. Tom will have to discuss this with Dr. H. We knew it could be one of this drug's possible side effects. The ringing in his ears has not gotten any better either.

Friday, April 1, 2005

Last night in bed, I could hear how labored Tom's breathing was and feared he has developed a respiratory infection. After a visit with the doctor, my fears were true, and Tom is on another antibiotic for the infection.

Sunday April 3, 2005

I am concerned about Tom. Even though Tom has not had treatment for two weeks, he is becoming more fatigued as the days go by. His hearing is still limited, but antibiotics seem to be helping. His breathing is a bit better but now as good as it can be.

I feel overwhelmed with taxes, FASA, SS disability filing and bills to pay on time. My sense of organization and thinking has not seemed to return as quickly as I need it to. Money is getting scarce, and we do not have enough from week to week to keep up. Tom is missing time from work which effects our income and prescriptions for both of us are costing from $300 - $400 a month, minimum.

Monday April 4, 2005

It is difficult to stay positive for Tom to help keep his spirits up. I still get very tired, and I am having difficulty dealing with depression. The Celexa is not helping as much as it had in the past.

I do not know what to think or how to feel about Tom's cancer. Mine went away. I was blessed and fortunate. Tom's cancer is much more life threatening. I want to assume that his will be cured as well, like mine.

I am afraid the reality is this will become a life-long struggle. If his cancer becomes controlled, I am afraid it will return, and he will have to have repeated treatments in an attempt to control it. Eventually, his body will give out and give in to the cancer.

The girls are struggling with college, both emotionally

and financially. I am going to the financial office and explain that Tom and I are both cancer patients and we are short of money.

Sadly, Tom and I have decided to sell the 1971 Mustang Fastback 351. We need the money and Tom said he could use the time we have been using to go to car shows to work on the 1972 Cuda. The Mustang has been a bonding experience for us. We spent two years restoring it and three years going to car shows together.

It is sad to see it go, but we do need the money.

Blood Cells - Chemotherapy
Wednesday, April 6, 2005

Tom's chemotherapy is postponed for this week. He has leucopenia, which is a severe decrease in his white blood cells. Decreased white blood cells make Tom vulnerable to infections.

Healthy blood cell counts are curial during radiation or chemotherapy treatments. There are three kinds of blood cells, White (WBC), Red (RBC), and Platelets (PLT).

White blood cells fight infections and within these cells are Lymphocytes, which are key cells of the immune system. It the white count becomes too low; a patient is vulnerable to serious infections. Red blood cells carry oxygen in the blood. Low levels of red cells cause paleness, fatigue, weakness, and dizziness. Platelets are important to help to stop bleeding. With low platelets, even the slightest cut can become difficult to stop from bleeding.

Tom is disappointed. I know he holds onto his hope through his chemotherapy treatments. I know he feels that if he misses a treatment his chance of survival decreases. This may be true, but with low blood counts, treatment would kill him faster than the cancer.

Thursday April 7, 2005

I went through a lot of depression yesterday. I just realized the reality that Tom could die. From what I read, lung cancer patients have about 12 – 18 months and with metastasized cancer to the brain, two and half years at the most. So, what I am to do? I do not want to think about my life without Tom. I feel guilty that I have survived my cancer and Tom may not survive his.

Sunday April 10, 2005

Today is my mom's birthday. I do not have the energy to drive all the way to Gordon to visit her.

I feel as though I am being pulled in too many directions. Tom wants so desperately to get taxes done, on-line selling, clean house and work on the Social Security disability forms. I cannot handle the pressure.

I know Tom is frustrated about missing his chemotherapy and worried he may miss the next one. I need to get away from all the pressure I feel right now. I need to forget for a while and relax.

Chemotherapy change
Tuesday April 12, 2005

At Tom's appointment today, Dr. H. reviewed Tom's hearing test results with him. He decided to stop the Cisplatin and substitute Cytoxan (Cyclophosphamide) instead. Further hearing loss may lessen with this drug, but it is not a guarantee.

Tom's white cells and platelet counts are within normal ranges, so Tom can continue with his chemotherapy tomorrow. He is continuing the antibiotic for his respiratory infection.

The more in-depth the realization that Tom is most likely going to die, the harder it is to accept my future life without him. It was not our plans. We were supposed to grow old together, like my parents who are married for over fifty-five years. They are like one. Tom and I were just becoming like one. After my treatments and the cure of my cancer, our lives had to chance to get better. Then five months later, boom, Tom receives a diagnosis of cancer.

It is not supposed to be that way. The two cancers in such a short time are draining our energy, our finances, and our future dreams. Now we must change our plans. Shorten them. I do not worry for me, but for Tom. I have a future and Tom may not.

I know that death is not unique. Married couples lose a partner every day. The dilemma is the road to Tom's demise with all the pain, hospitals, treatments, and bills. Added to this, I am not physically sound, and I feel a need to hide this from Tom. There is absolutely no normalcy in our lives at all, none.

Cycle Three – Chemotherapy
Wednesday, April 13, 2005 - Chemotherapy

Tom had his session one of cycle three with the new chemotherapy drug, Cytoxan, today. The nurse had some difficulty finding a usable vein for Tom's IV. After a couple of tries, she was able to get the IV inserted. The IV will stay in place for the next three days while Tom receives his treatments.

Amongst all the turmoil and chaos in our lives, a little rainbow was born. My niece Christina had a little girl today and named her Elizabeth.

Thursday, April 14, 2005 - Chemotherapy

We watched movies and TV most of the day of Tom's session two of cycle three. We do not talk much while we are sitting, but it is important to me that I stay during Tom's treatment. Tom asked me to go and find something to do and not to spend all day sitting with him. I assured him there was no place I would rather be, than sitting next to him. He accepted that.

I finished our income taxes and put them in the mail making that one less stress I had to worry about for now.

A rainbow appeared once again today. My niece Sandra May gave birth to a little girl and named her Cypress.

Friday, April 15, 2005 – Chemotherapy

Tom is feeling tired today. It is the third session of cycle three and I am certain that the chemo drugs are taking their toll on Tom's blood and body. He still wants to go to the car show at UW Stout tomorrow.

Sunday, April 16, 2005

Today was the first car show of the year for us. It was at UW Stout in Menomonie. We brought the 351 Mustang and put a "For Sale" sign on it. Everyone was curious as to why we were selling it. We explained that I had just gotten through with cancer treatment and Tom was now in treatment. We needed the money. There were a few inquiries, but no one serious.

It was good to see some old car show friends, but by early afternoon, Tom was tired and ready to go home. I was grateful that he was not too tired to drive since I never learned how to handle the clutch on the Mustang.

I did not realize that this was the last car show Tom, and I would bring a car too again.

Tuesday, April 18, 2005

I am continuing to use drops in Tom's ears in an effort to give him some release, but the drops no longer seem to help.

Thursday April 21, 2005

I am trying to clean the house from all the clutter that has accumulated over the past months. I worked on some file cabinets and tried to organize all the medical bills we have. I do not understand why Tom and I each must have our own account with the same service provider. Now, instead of sending one payment to cover both of us, we are required to send two payments, one each for every medical service we have received. I am writing 10 checks a month just to cover minimums on two accounts each.

I do not know where the money is going to come from to cover all the bills.

I have no clue where Tom is as far as his treatments. I know he is done with radiation and has one more three-day chemotherapy session. He seems to be doing well except for the hearing loss.

I am in such turmoil about his dying. When will it happen? Will we have some indication that is will be soon? I was thinking about working on Tom's picture memory board because deep inside I doubt that he will survive. If he does not, the last thing I am going to want to do is go through pictures to organize in remembrance of him.

It is almost unbearable to be around Tom these days.

There has been too much disappointment too soon with his treatments. We have been without the internet for over a week now. The internet keeps Tom occupied so he does not have to think so much. It is also a resource for selling. We still have many motorcycle and car parts to sell as well many electronics. Without the internet, we cannot sell, and the bills get overwhelming. When Tom misses work for treatments, his check is lower and there is not enough to make ends meet.

Friday April 22, 2005

Tom and I were talking today about fear. We fear what we do not know or understand. Before my treatments, I was afraid of what I did not know or understand. I did not know how radiation and chemotherapy would affect my body, my attitude, or my tumor.

Experience helps to ease fear. I survived what I feared. It is over and I am still here. If I had to go through it again, I would still have a degree of fear. Not of the treatment itself, but of surviving it since I came so close to dying the first time around.

I asked Tom if he was afraid before he started treatment.

He said, "Yes, because I thought it would be like yours. I thought I would be in a lot of pain and be sick like you were."

I admitted to him that I thought the same thing. I am incredibly grateful that his treatments are not as radical and full of severe side effects as mine was. His hearing loss is bad enough.

A few days ago, Tom kept saying he wished his hair were back. I asked him why it was so important.

He said, "I'm bald. Everyone at work knows I have cancer. They avoid me and don't talk to me very much anymore."

"My boss and I used to have talks in his office. He doesn't do that anymore."

My heart just broke. He was like a child coming home from school after being teased and rejected on the playground.

People do treat you differently when you have cancer. Since I did not lose my hair, it was not as obvious. Some friends of mine who knew I had cancer treated me differently. They stop calling or asking to do things together.

I guess when someone has cancer, it is a reminder to others that we are mortal, and we may die from our cancer. Nevertheless, many people survive and as I have said before, the support we get from others is as important as the treatments.

Saturday April 23, 2005

I have been trying to get Tom to discuss the future in the event his does not survive. He is having a difficult time with being terminal. We did decide that it was time to make a will. I want to discuss Tom's wishes, just in case he doesn't survive, but I didn't know how to approach it so I will let it go for now.

I was thinking that a memorial and the internment should be in Gordon. We met in Gordon, married at St Anthony's Church in Gordon, and had our children baptized there. However, that is a long way for his friends and co-workers to go for a funeral. This is why I wanted to discuss it with Tom. I do not know what it is he would want.

I do not want to deal with it after he is gone, especially since I am not sure of his wishes.

Sandy and I talked about Tom being terminal. I do not want to accept it. I know I must come to terms with it. I am more concerned about Tom coming to terms with it. It is happening to him. It will affect the rest of us, but he is the one whose life will end.

We all are going to die. His advantage (if you can call it that) is that he knows approximately when. He could have the opportunity to conclude his life on his terms. He could have the opportunity to conclude things he needs to take care of. He can say his goodbyes and make any amends he feels necessary. I know he has to deal with the anxiety that he has been told he is going to die. Since he still will not talk about it, I do not know about his true thoughts.

Unlike people who die suddenly, without warning, he is pre-warned. What he does with this information is his choice. I want the end of his life to be more than just "four walls".

Second Opinion

Monday April 25, 2005

Tom has been talking about getting a second opinion about his cancer and wanted me to check and see if he could get into Mayo Clinic in Rochester. I spoke with a doctor at Mayo Clinic, and he said we could come down for Tom's evaluation right after his last chemotherapy sessions. This session would be from May 4 to May 6.

The Mayo doctor said in his opinion that Tom's cancer was very serious, and he has only about nine months left. He said the evaluation would tell us more. I did not tell Tom what the doctor had said of his timeline. I decided to let the doctor tell him once we got there.

Later, Phillip and I talked about a family vacation. I had thought about a cruise, but with Tom's treatments, I would not feel comfortable about his health. I do know that I want to go to Oregon for a visit. I want to go and see Crater Lake with Tom. Ever since I was in grade school and we had studied it, I wanted to go. It is important to me to share it with Tom.

Tuesday April 26, 2005

Tom is going to Mayo Clinic on May 10 and 11. Strange how it ended up being May 10 as that is my birthday. They will evaluative his condition and give us a second opinion. His boss suggested Tom go to Mayo, so this should make him happy that Tom took his suggestion.

There is a lot of prep to do before we can go. I have a list of six items to do. Guess I will go finish Tom's Social Security Disability application now.

Thursday April 28, 2005

Tom started an antibiotic, Cipro, today for respiratory infection.

Friday April 29, 2005

I feel extremely overwhelmed today. I am trying to contact everyone on my Mayo list, but it is not as easy as it seems. The biopsy from the hospital in St Paul is working out to be the most difficult. I must physically go and get the sample. We need to complete a release form as well.

Tom's white count is very low. If his blood count does not come up, they will postpone his chemo again and that may goof up the Mayo Clinic appointment.

Sandy and I talked today. She realizes that Tom's days are numbered. So do I. How do you make someone's last days on earth enjoyable and worthwhile? Tom will not talk about it because then he would have to deal with the fact that he is dying.

Sunday May 1, 2005

It snowed today. About one quarter inch of snow stayed on the ground. We listed the Mustang on the internet. We have had many questions about it. I am sure it will sell. I made some more jewelry to sell on the internet and with the motorcycle parts; we will be able to pay for our prescriptions this month. There are so many things going on all at once and I feel stressed by it all.

Monday May 2, 2005

I was able to get Tom's biopsy sample to take with us to Mayo Clinic. That is one less thing on my list.

Tom acceptance to go to Mayo Clinic is because they want him to participate in their Lung Cancer study. I think if his being in the study can help with lung cancer research, it is an incredibly good thing. His contribution to the health of other people who are also fighting lung cancer could end up being valuable information someday.

My mind will not stop going over things, so I am not able to sleep. The Cipro is making Tom dizzy and tired. Combined with chemo, he is very exhausted. He keeps going to work. I do not know how he does it.

I spoke with my friend, Kathy, about Mayo Clinic. She was surprised Tom got in so fast. She said she was surprised that we got in at all. She also said that the waiting list is usually a minimum of 12 weeks. Tom only had to wait 2 weeks for an appointment.

I hope he has his chemo this week. I would hate to goof up his opportunity to go to Mayo.

There are motorcycle parts all over the house. We own

so much junk. I need to be very dedicated about listing on the internet. I need to clean all this stuff out of here and make some money while we are at it.

I am still having bloody stools. The blood is on the outside with a lot of mucus. My lungs still hurt, and I am still coughing. I slept from 10:30 last night until 11:00 this morning. I still feel very tired though.

Tuesday May 3, 2005

Tom went to work today. He is still feeling poorly. I hope he gets his chemo tomorrow.

Every time I look up lung cancer information, I cringe at the words, one-year survival. It is very difficult to imagine Tom will be dead in a matter of months.

It is inevitable that he will die within a year. I cannot stand the thought of that. He is my life, and he is my best friend. He is my companion. What will I do without him? He is like a perfect pair of boots. I do not want him to be gone.

Cycle Four – Chemotherapy
Wednesday May 4, 2005 - Chemotherapy

Tom's white cells went from 1600 to 4600 in a week. He was on Cipro and even though it made him sick, it did what it was supposed to do. He had session one of cycle four today. The nurse had to try a few times to get the IV in, but she was successful.

Now we are on schedule for Mayo Clinic. I need to check out a hotel room for overnight. Many hotels accommodate Mayo Clinic patients while they visit the clinic.

Tom looks peaky today. He is pale and his eyes seem glazed appearing. Tom seems to be suffering. He has pain in his joints and his side still hurts from bumping into the dumpster two weeks ago.

Thursday, May 5, 2005 - Chemotherapy

Tom had session two of cycle four today. His blood veins were better and the IV went in easily. I am happy for that. When things do not go smoothly, Tom becomes stressed. He does not need any additional stress.

Financial Estate Will
Friday, May 6, 2005- Chemotherapy
After Tom had session three of cycle four, we met with an attorney to write our wills. It was eerie to sit with an attorney, listing our assets and deciding what will happen to them if either Tom or I died. We created two Wills, one for Tom and one for me.

There are advantages to having a Will if you own any type of assets such as a house, investments, stocks, or other financial aspects. A Will assures that your final wishes will be carried out, and things will be left to the people of your choice. The laws vary from state to state, but often, the state will decide what will happen to your assets if you die without a Will. A Will is important at any point of your life once you accumulate assets, so creating a Will even without a terminal illness is important for anyone.

Second Anal Ultra-sound - Rita
Monday May 9, 2005
I can see Tom change with each passing day. His short-term memory is very poor. His sense of sorting or finding something is getting worse with each day. He cannot comprehend simple directions, which has become more difficult for him.

I sit here and wonder how I feel as I watch and care for Tom as he is dying. It is hard to realize that a process is happening right in front of me, and I am powerless to change it.

I had my second anal ultra-sound today. I am still negative for cancer. It would be exciting news and I would like to celebrate, but with Tom's condition, I cannot celebrate.

Tomorrow will be a very important day for him. There will be many tests and then the doctor's opinion of his prognosis. I am praying there is still hope for him.

Since Tom and I would be in Rochester for my birthday, Phillip surprised me with a cake and some awesome colored flame candles. He also bought me a bottle of wine from Sonoma

County.

C

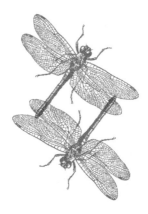

CHAPTER 9 - TOM'S CONTINUED TREATMENTS

Mayo Clinic Experience
Tuesday May 10, 2005

We pushed hard this morning to get Mayo Clinic on time. I wanted to leave by 6:30 a.m. but we did not leave until 7:10 a.m. Tom was slow in getting started. It was a ninety-two-mile trip.

We had no idea what the Mayo Clinic in Rochester, Minnesota was like. We had never been there, making the apprehension we felt, escalate.

I was first impressed with the vastness of the insides of the various buildings. We had to ask for directions as soon as we entered the Mayo Building. There were people in every nook and cranny to offer help. If someone was standing around with an empty expression, indicating they were either lost or confused, someone was at their side immediately, offering help.

When we finally found our way to the admissions area, my first impression of the check-in system had a remarkable resemblance to the check-in area of the airport.

At the time we registered, we received a complete schedule of Tom's tests, times, and their locations. This pre-planning made it quite easy to get from one area of the clinic to another with enough time for each test.

At 9:30 a.m., our first stop was for blood tests.

The next test was at 10:15 and was an MRI. The handout we received completely explained what an MRI was; the procedure and how long it would take.

Things have been going well here, as it is highly organized and efficient. We were getting in a little early with each test. It is hard to spend so much time waiting, but I have a feeling I had better get used to it.

At noon, Tom had a CT done. Again, we received an informative handout about what a CT was and how long it took.

After completing the CT, we were free to go for the rest of the day.

We are going to stay at the nearby casino tonight. Lindalee and Jeff are going to meet us there so we can celebrate my birthday.

We must be back at the clinic by 8:30 in the morning to review all the test results.

Wednesday, May 11, 2005

We met with a clinic doctor who reviewed the results of the tests with us. The review of the MRI impressed me. The doctor showed us the "slices" of imaging they had done and explained each one as we viewed it. The MRI indicated that the brain tumors had decreased in size and number. That was encouraging.

The tumor in the lung had also decreased in size as well. The tumor in the Adrenal gland remained unchanged, which was good news since it had not increased in size.

The doctor told us that Dr. H. was following a treatment plan that they would have used at Mayo and encourage Tom to continue seeing him. She explained that they would be obtaining Tom's progress information of his treatments from Dr. H. and will add this information to their research studies of lung cancer.

I was pleased to hear that Dr. H. was right on with his

treatments for Tom and that Tom could be greatly confident under his care in the future. They assured us that Dr. H. would receive the restaging results for his review.

Monday, May 16, 2005

Tom is showing signs of Raynaud's type symptoms resulting in cold fingers and toes. Raynaud's disease is a vascular disorder that causes intermittent interruption of blood flow to the extremities. The affected body part may turn white or blue and feel cold and numb until circulation improves.

Tom's blood counts are low. The chemotherapy is taking its toll on his blood counts, which in turn take their toll on Tom. He is showing signs of being tired more often than when he is not.

Thursday May 19, 2005

Tom and I have been married 26 years today. What a fabulous accomplishment. I smile every time I think of our wedding day. It was the best party ever!

Dr. H. had not yet received the information from Mayo Clinic by the time Tom went in today for his appointment. Tom and I explained the tests results the best we could remember. Dr. H. will continue Tom's treatment with chemotherapy.

It is amazing how many people have cancer and how many are cancer survivors. It seems like cancer does touch everyone's life in one form or another.

For today, it was a good day. Tom's recent tests showed hope and we are happy to celebrate another year together. I made us a romantic dinner with candles, but Tom was not hungry and went to bed early.

Friday May 20, 2005

I spent the day with the girls in Menomonie today. We went to lunch and shopped for art supplies. The store was having its annual clearance sale. It was a good time for art majors to get some inexpensive supplies.

Unfortunately, I had some bowel problems on my way home, had to take a bath, and wash my jeans. It was frustrating since the lack of bowel control is getting more frequent. I am still dealing with my bladder control problems and find it frustrating to have to be concerned about my bowels as well. I have begun to use protective under garments more often now, especially if I am going to go out for any length of time.

Having to use protective undergarments at my age is very emotional and I have not learned how to deal with it yet.

Monday May 23, 2005

I have been on the phone most of the day with medical services that want their money. It has been difficult to make ends meet. We still have not sold the 1971 Mustang yet. We had an offer, but the person changed his mind at the last minute. We will have to try again.

Cycle Five – Chemotherapy
Wednesday, May 25, 2005

Tom had session one of cycle five today. Tom is feeling better today. Still very tired but holding onto the positive attitude he obtained from his recent tests results.

Thursday, May 26, 2005 - Chemotherapy

Today while I was sitting with Tom, I wondered about all the people who sit in chemotherapy by themselves. Even though I am mostly sitting here, I think it gives Tom comfort and the knowledge that I am supporting him. Today was session two of cycle five.

Friday, May 27, 2005 - Chemotherapy

Today was session three of cycle five. Tom has had so much chemotherapy by now. I am amazed that he tolerates it so well. I know he would not complain if it did bother him. He just keeps pushing on each day and holds onto the hope that he will survive his cancer and we can continue with our lives. It is a good thing to have hope.

Wednesday, June 1, 2005

Tom's left foot is showing signs of slight swelling. If it continues to get worse, he will need to go to the doctor and have it checked. There is also a slight rash on his foot, and it is starting to swell. I asked him to go to the doctor as soon as possible. He said he would.

Monday, June 6, 2005

My dad is seventy-five years old today. A long time to live, and hopefully there will be a lot more. I am hoping that a cure for Tom will come along so I can look forward to his seventy-fifth birthday.

On one hand, I see the reality that Tom may die and on the other, I keep hoping that a cure for his cancer is found. The reality part allows me to prepare for his death, yet the possibility for a cure is my hope. There is always hope even amidst the reality. There is always hope up until the day Tom dies.

My stress level is at an all-time high. I have headaches all the time and four or five bowel movements per day. Tom is getting more tired by the day. He is about at his limit. The other day he said he did not want to work anymore. Tom has always enjoyed his work. It fulfilled his need for creativity and gave him a strong sense of accomplishment. I was surprised by his statement, but I was also surprised that he has worked this long while in treatment.

Then he tentatively sold the other Mustang we own, the 429 Mustang, for $500 less than what we paid for it. I asked him why.

He said, "Because I'm dying."

I was surprised to hear Tom say those words aloud. I wish he had more faith that he could beat it. If he does not believe that he can survive, he will not. He started smoking again but does not have the emotional strength to quit permanently. Even though he has reduced a lot, it would be best if he quit all together.

He has no ambition lately. The problem is he wants to do things through me. I have already taken over his trash and dump duties. Phillip has taken over cutting the grass and yard work. I have been doing the car restorations as best as I can.

I am having my own physical problems. I am having frequent and loose stools with lots of intestinal pain and cramps. I am also having some vaginal discharge. Tom and I are trying to resume a healthy sex life, but it is extremely painful for me, and I have not, and will not tell Tom. It is the only degree of what I can call normal in our lives. If he does not know about my pain level, it will be ok with me. It may get better.

My frequency of fatigue is coming back, and I am experiencing depression again.

Tuesday, June 7, 2005

My concern for Tom is increasing. He seems to have given up. The only thing he wants is for me to do internet selling all the time. I do have other things to do, but he cannot see that.

His left foot is still swollen, and the rash is worse. He also has a nasty wood tick bite on his stomach. He made an appointment to see a doctor tomorrow.

He gets blood drawn tomorrow. I think he needs to take have his anti-depressant adjusted. He is so very depressed, but I can understand why he is this way.

Wednesday, June 8, 2005

Tom is tired these days. He has no interest in anything. He comes home and sits in front of the computer all night. His blood count is down, only 1500 (white). He has staph infection on his foot and at the site of the tick bite. He is on an antibiotic for the infection and an allergy medication to help relieve the itching on both his foot and the tick bite.

I am sure these medications are contributing to his fatigue. He is still working every day, except the ones when he has chemotherapy. He stopped saying he did not want to work anymore.

Friday, June 10, 2005

Tom stayed home from work because he was too tired. The antibiotic for the staph infection seems to be helping. His foot still burns but the swelling has gone down. The inflammation from the tick bite on his stomach is gone as well.

Lately Tom is like a child sometimes. He will be doing something and forget what he was doing. He has difficulty following directions. His comprehension is poor. He is tired and depressed. I cannot even imagine how hard it is for him at work. I am grateful that his work understands. He has done so many good things for his company that I am sure they are showing appreciation. Being the Engineering Manager must prove to be very difficult for Tom these days.

Cycle Six – Chemotherapy
Wednesday, June 15, 2005

Today was session one cycle six of Tom's chemotherapy. His veins are weakening again. It took a few tries this time to get an IV inserted. I think Tom should have considered a port, but he said he is still not interested in the surgery to have it done.

Thursday June 16, 2005

Tomorrow is Tom's last chemo for now. This is the sixth three-day session. He gets a CT next week. I had one yesterday. I got cramps and the diarrhea. I am still having cramps today.

Tom and I were talking yesterday and out of nowhere, he said he wanted to be cremated. I wanted to ask him what to do with his ashes, but that is all he would say about it, and I did not pursue it any further. I was surprised he said anything at all about dying.

Friday June 17, 2005 - Chemotherapy

Today is the third session of cycle six and Tom will be done with chemotherapy for a while. I am happy for that. The treatments have been taking their toll on him. He continues to miss work on the days he has chemo and the other days at work are a real struggle for him. I know at times; he puts his head on his desk and sleeps. No one bothers him.

Saturday June 18, 2005

The Boss 351 Mustang was sold today. Yet another change in our lives. The changes are happening so fast that they make my head whirl. We still have the 429 Mustang and Tom doesn't seem as anxious to sell it.

Monday June 20, 2005

I asked Tom how he felt today. He said he did not feel sick but did not feel well. He said everything hurts and his whole body ached. He also told me he felt impatient and apprehensive.

He said, "I just want things to go back to normal. Not being able to hear is the hardest. I am tired all the time and I fall asleep at my desk. How embarrassing. They are keeping me around. I do not accomplish anything. I want things back the way they used to be."

I felt helpless to comfort him. I need a plan.

I called Sandy to tell her how sad Tom was.

She and I began concocting a vacation plan for Tom and me to Oregon. Sandy and Larry have been all over Oregon and have some great ideas. I told her my priority is to see Crate Lake. We tentatively planned on July 24 – August 2, 2005, for the trip.

The plan we came up with was to get to Oregon first, then go to the coast, Crater Lake, Reno, and Tahoe, and then back to Portland along the coastline. Tom has never been to Oregon, and I know he will love it.

I am going to try to talk Tom into taking two weeks off. I cannot see trying to do it in one week. Tom needs something to look forward to and I hope this will do that. A trip would be good for both of us.

I talked to Tom about the trip. He was worried about the money. I told him that the money from the Mustang sale would be enough to pay some medical bills and to take the trip.

I was sad to think the Mustang was sold and that the car movers will be here Thursday. I am not looking forward to Thursday, and I know it is breaking Tom's heart to have to sell the Mustang.

He so loves classic cars. I am glad that I enjoyed restoring them with him. It gave us a lot of quality time together. We would check over restoration specs and make them happen.

Tuesday, June 21, 2005

My stress level is increasing again. With the stress of the Mustang being sold and the problems with Tom's health, I find it all very difficult to deal with.

Tom is getting more difficult to live with by no fault of his own. He is irritable and depressed. His hearing loss is bothering him very much. Hearing aids will not improve his hearing so there is nothing else to do.

He tells me that I cannot imagine what it is like. He is right. I cannot imagine it. Yet he cannot imagine how difficult it is for me to have the TV so loud that it gets on my nerves. On the other hand, when he speaks so softly that I have to ask him to repeat himself and he gets angry with me for asking him to repeat.

His tolerance for everything is low. I was talking about the poor condition of the freezer, and he became extremely angry and yelled, "We'll get a new one". All I asked was if replacing the door magnetic seals was possible.

The basement shower leaks and is causing mold in the shower. The basement toilet is broken and the septic needs attention. The Tahoe and the Honda need repair and so on. I do not dare bring any of this up to him for fear of his reaction. He normally would be on top of any repairs that are needed but under the circumstances, it is understandable why he is not.

Wednesday, June 22, 205

I talked to Tom about the trip to Oregon. He was not excited. That is depressing to me. I just do not know how to make life any better for him. He is just concerned about money and concerned about what will happen to things after he is gone. Personally, I think if he were so concerned about any of it, he would have had life insurance, and life and casualty insurance on the house. Now it is too late for either.

If I cannot maintain this house, I will have to sell it. It is not paid for yet. I do not like thinking about where and how to live. It seems like it would not matter where I live if Tom is gone. If I am careful with money and have a job, I will be OK. I am not interested in what my life will be like after he is gone.

I continue to worry about my cancer coming back. With insufficient medical insurance, I would not be able to have treatments.

Life is a strange existence. Some people have good lives, and some people live lives of turmoil. Our lives are somewhere in between. Cancer has really screwed our lives up. It has robbed us of our dreams and our health. We are like strangers again. Since Tom diagnosis, my recovery has become non-existent to Tom.

It is as if the clock stopped on my cancer and began again with his. He seems to think I am 100% and expects me to have my normal energy level and able to do all the things I used to be able. I am down to 130 pounds from 150 pounds. The weight loss seems to be affecting my energy level as well. I just do not have the energy as I did one and a half years ago.

Tom is drinking again. He seems to think he is guaranteed to die, so he does not seem to care. I am afraid he does not care it he lives or dies.

I remember being there. It was in October in the middle of my radiation and chemo treatments. It seemed like so much work to make it from day to day. I was so exhausted, and life did not seem real anymore. Family and friends encouraged me to go on. That is my new task for Tom, to give him daily encouragement. Just because, as of today, he is terminal, that could change in the near future. Once again that is what I call hope. Hope until it is to late, the day he dies. I just need to help him feel that hope as well.

I remember thinking to myself after my diagnosis that I could handle anything that came my way. I had my husband, family and friends for support, so I felt well-armed for any situation that arouse. When Tom received his diagnosis of cancer five months later, I was convinced that I was not prepared for a journey where both Tom and I had to battle not only our own cancer, but each other's as well.

I was facing many issues I was not prepared to face. Feelings of being overwhelmed surface daily as I learned new aspects dealing with cancer. There are many times when I feel defeated and all alone with my thoughts and feelings.

I am living from both sides of cancer. As a survivor, I want to feel the joy of being one, but the cloud of Tom's cancer looms so intensely above us, I feel guilt for being a survivor instead of joy.

I realize now that my previous role as a cancer patient is having an enormous impact as we face Tom's cancer. The experience has served as an important resource to provide strength to Tom, which will allow him to die with dignity. My love for Tom and his tremendous tenacity and determination to survive, has given me strength I did not realize I had.

I hope as the months pass, I can continue to grow in strength so that Tom realizes that he is not alone.

Thursday, June 23, 2005

The truck came today for the Boss 351 Mustang. They could not make it up our drive, so we had to take the Mustang to a flat area down the road. Tom walked all around the car with such loving affection. It held many memories for us and many dreams. In a few moments, those dreams would drive off forever.

I took a picture of Tom standing next to the car before it left. I could see the sadness in his eyes. It seemed like just another day of disappointments for him. I hated to see the car go too since it meant so much to me in memories as well.

Friday, June 24, 2005

The doctor put Tom on Wellbutrin to help with his depression and I do not think it mixes well with chemotherapy.

Monday, June 27, 2005

Tom had a CT with contrast today.

My emotions are confusing lately. I cannot view death as a horrid thing that happens to everyone or I would not be able to handle Tom's death. I do view it as a severe loss. Yet, I cannot view death as "it happens to everyone" because then I would be insensitive to death, including my own.

I feel like I am in limbo. Is Tom going to live? Do we play wait and see? Do we accept that he is going to die and go from there? Do we say he is not going to die and not change anything and not prepare for it?

Do I plan my future as though I will be alone or plan as though Tom will be around? It is such a dilemma and makes my heart ache when I think about it. My daughters told me if I accept that Tom is going to die, then I am giving up hope. I do not agree.

With each passing day, I hope a cure is found. With each passing day, I hope that Tom will have the strength to be here as long as it takes for that cure. However, with each passing day I also look at the reality that without that cure, he will die.

Tuesday, June 28, 2005

Tom and I had appointments today with Dr. H. today. I could see the disappointment in Tom's eyes when he did not hear the word "cure". Instead, he heard "hopefully we won't have to do chemo again until November or December". Dr. H. explained that the reason for delaying chemotherapy was that the lung masses did show some decrease in size in several areas. He did say however, that he had a concern about two tiny cysts in the caudate lobe in the liver.

He once again spoke to Tom that there is a high likelihood that the cancer will start continued growth within the next few months. He also reminded Tom that death could occur in the upcoming months.

It seems so scary to realize that Tom is going to die. It is a matter of when. We are all going to die someday, but it is so different when it is established with a timeline.

I continue to have both bladder and bowel incontinence. I have a diagnosis of radiation cystitis and radiation proctitis. This means that I have inflammation and damage to both the bladder and sigmoid colon and rectum. I also have another bladder infection.

Tom finally decided that we should go on the trip to Oregon. I am happy that he said yes. It will be good for him to relax and enjoy himself. He does not have chemotherapy for the next two months at least, so he can afford the time to go. Getting his vacation time off work was no problem and everyone at his work is excited that he is going on a well-deserved vacation.

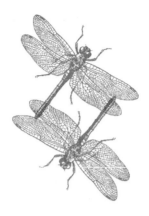

APTER 10 - CONTINUED HOPE

Thursday, June 30, 2005

Tom's hair is growing back. It is just fuzz, but his mustache is back, and he has managed to grow a small Go-T. I know having his mustache back is important to him. I cannot remember when he did not have one.

Saturday, July 2, 2005

Even though Tom was tired, he wanted to go to Gordon for the Fourth of July. It is strange to think we were not bringing the Mustang to Gordon for the parade. Last year our car took the People Choice Award. Tom and my dad would drive the car in the parade and my dad would throw the candy. Tom always managed to get a few wheel squeals done before the end of the parade route.

Even though I was feeling tired, I did as I have for the past twelve years, I helped with the brat sales. The money from the sales goes to finance the annual Halloween Party for the town's children.

Monday July 4, 2005

I went to the Miller Family reunion in Siren, Wisconsin today. Tom was so tired from the trip to Gordon that he decided to stay home. Phillip and Rachel went also. It was an enjoyable

get together.
Tuesday, July 5, 2005

Tom did miss taking the Mustang to Gordon. Logically, selling it was for the best, I guess. We are not going to car shows anymore and we really needed the money. The money was enough to catch up with most of the medical bills and enough left over to spend on a vacation to Oregon.

I know I should probably save the money to pay medical bills, but I am afraid that if we do not go to Oregon now, we will never get to go. I do not know how much time Tom has left, and I do not want to lose the opportunity to do something fun for him.

Wednesday July 6, 2005

Sandy and I spent hours today talking back and forth making plans for our trip. We mapped the miles and activities to determine how much we could squeeze into two weeks.

Monday, July 11, 2005

I went to my appointment with the urologist today. My CT results showed some thickening of the bladder wall. He started me on Vesicare to help reduce the urgency to void. I go back in a month for a cystourethroscopy to examine the inside of the bladder.

Friday, July 8, 2005

Tom got tests results from a recent CT of his abdomen, and it was positive for liver metastases. I feel helpless when I realize that the cancer is going to win. Tom is fighting so hard to retain his life, but the odds are stacking up against him.

Thursday, July 14, 2005

I am getting excited for our trip to Oregon. I have been there a few times to visit my sister, Sandy, but Tom has never been there. I am excited to share places I have been, and even more excited to share Carter Lake with Tom. I want Tom to start doing things that bring him joy so he can spend his remaining days looking at life from another perspective other than waiting for death.

Oregon Trip
Friday, July 22, 2005

I managed to take care of the luggage when we got the airport. I hate flying so I turned to Tom for courage. He finds it funny that I am so afraid of flying. When we lived in Kentucky, he was working on his pilot's license.

Sandy and Larry were at the airport in Oregon to meet us. It was nice to fly non-stop. We went out for dinner in Portland and then went over our travel plans. It is exciting to think we can spend a few weeks just relaxing.

Saturday July 23, 2005

Tom slept very well last night and had energy and interest to see Portland. It just so happened that the annual beer festival was taking place in the park today so we went to it. It was not that exciting since none of us were in the mood to taste beer. We walked along the Columbia Gorge and enjoyed seeing all the boats.

We went to Saturday market. All the artists and their wares were impressive. After lunch, Larry took us to a liquidator outlet store and Tom, and I found some fun gifts to take back home with us.

Sunday, July 24, 2005

Rising early, we packed the car for our trip around Oregon and surrounding states. A few planned stops along the way were to the casinos. Tom really enjoyed going to casinos and rooms at most casino is more reasonable than most hotels.

Our first touring stop was Crater Lake. I do not think I have ever seen such beautiful blue water in my whole life. I was windy and the breeze felt good on such a hot day.

We had hotel reservations in Klamath Falls, OR so we piled back in the van and headed south. It was dusk when we neared Klamath Falls and had to drive several miles along the lake. Unfortunately, tiny bugs were hatching by the millions.

The air was so full of tiny bugs; it was like a misty rain. The bugs clung to the windshield, the antenna, and the entire front of the van. Larry stopped wiping them off the windshield because the wipers just smeared them along the glass.

We found our hotel late, bugs and all and checked in. When I first walked to the bathroom, I had the sensation that I was walking downhill. I figured it was my imagination, so I did not mention it. When I walked from the bathroom the bed area, I felt as though I were walking uphill. I still did not say anything. I did not want anyone to think I was going crazy!

Then one by one, they had the same experience. We all began to laugh. The floor was sloping downward. Maybe it was upward. Either way, the floor was not level. The next morning at breakfast, we asked about the curious floor. It seems there was an earthquake and that is what happened to the floor. Once we were outside, we looked carefully at the buildings and their state of different crookedness made us laugh. We did; however, decide we would never stay in a hotel in that area again.

After leaving the hotel, we went to a gas station and spent the next half hour scrubbing and scraping bugs off the car and out of the grille.

Monday, July 25 and 26, 2005

The next two nights will be spent in Sparks, Nevada. Sandy and Larry had a time-share in Sparks, so we were able to save on hotel costs. Tom was so excited. There were so many casinos all within walking distance. We had a great time jumping from casino to casino.

Shortly before we sat down to eat; Larry discovered that he had lost his billfold. In a panic, we went back to the casino's we had visited, and had no luck finding it.

We eat our supper while Larry made a list of the places, he had to call to report missing charge cards and license.

Tuesday, July 26, 2005

The next morning before doing anything else, Larry spent over an hour on the phone cancelling his cards and reporting his loss.

We ate a nice breakfast and headed to Tahoe. Larry felt naked without any ID. He said he was a "nobody".

Lake Tahoe was beautiful, and we enjoyed watching the boats. We drove around the area and saw many beautiful things. On the way back to Sparks, we stopped at a few casinos in Reno. Tom got tired so we called it an early night.

We cooked a nice meal in our room and enjoyed each other's company.

Wednesday, July 27, 2005

The next morning when we were packing to leave, sitting under Larry's black fan, was his billfold. When he flipped it onto the dresser, it fell under the fan! Imagine that.

On our way to Anderson, CA, we stopped at a grocery and bought an exceptionally large bag of cherries. We had some apples and oranges and dined on a fruit snack as we drove. As we approached California, we saw a sign that said we could not bring any fruits or vegetables into the state.

We looked at our fruit stash and laughed. We spent the next hour eating our fruit. When we got to the state entrance station, the attendant waved us through. We were surprised they did not want to check us for fruit. We laughed about it for the next hour.

Tom was having a good time and it was nice to see him enjoying himself. Occasionally I would ask him how he felt, and he would say "Good".

On the way, we passed through Lassen National Park. It was full of geyser, trees, and even snow. Tom got out of the car, walked up a small hill, and threw snowballs at us while wearing a t-shirt and shorts. It was fun.

Thursday, July 28, 2005

We stayed at the casino in Canyonville, OR. Tom was tired by this time, so he slept a few hours when we got there. After he woke, we ate and gambled for a while. Tom seemed like his old self. He gets so excited when he is playing. I just loved it.

Friday, July 29, 2005

We left the casino and as we were driving to our hotel in Lincoln City, we drove along the coast through Coos Bay. Passing through the town, Tom saw a sign for deep-sea fishing. He got excited and said he wanted to do that.

We stopped by the charter office and made inquiries. They did not have a waiting list and it was first come first serve. If we were interested, we had to be at the dock by 6:00 a.m. Tom was extremely interested.

Once we got to the hotel, Tom expressed his concerns about getting cold. Even with the warm summer air, Tom was cold more often than not. Sandy and I left Tom and Larry at the hotel and went coat shopping. We found a nice, insulated coat at a discount store and hoped it would help.

Saturday, July 30, 2005

We dropped Tom and Larry off at the dock and took pictures as their boat shimmed off across the ocean waters, I was concerned about Tom getting cold, but he had on enough clothes for a mid-west winter's day.

We went back six hours later. The expression on Tom's face was like a child on Christmas morning. He showed us his basket of fish and smiled. It was great to see him enjoy such a special event. He had never been ocean fishing and I am grateful he got the opportunity.

He was exhausted but happy. We took their fish and headed back to Sandy and Larry's house in Beaverton.

Sunday, July 31, 2005

Since Tom was getting tired from all the traveling, we decided to have a leisurely day. We drove up to Washington State and looked at the mountains as we drove by. We stopped for a light lunch and went back to the house.

Larry had a seafood dinner all planned for us and started getting it ready. Sandy and Larry's children and grandchildren joined us for dinner. It was good to see all of them.

Monday, August 1, 2005

Tom was feeling tired and was anxious to get home. The plane trip went well and once we arrived home, Tom went to sleep.

Tuesday, August 2, 2005

Tom went back to work today. He feels tired but is concerned to get his work done.

TIA (Transient Ischemic Attack) – Tom
Monday, August 8, 2005

Tom ended up in the ER today. At first, his boss called me and asks me to come and get Tom from work. He did not say what was wrong. Before I got to the plant, he called again and asked me to meet them at the hospital.

I went to emergency and found Tom there. My heart had been pounding all the way into town. He was sitting there, and I was relieved that he had not died.

Tom had a TIA-mini stroke. After completing a CT of the chest, brain, abdomen, and pelvis, and he was allowed to go home. Tom slept for the rest of the afternoon.

TIA (Transient Ischemic Attack) or commonly known as a mini stroke occurs when the brain does not get enough blood and oxygen. In Tom's case, the brain tumors are causing constriction on the blood vessels of the brain. Constricted blood vessels or clots are the primary cause of TIA.

Symptoms of TIA are weakness or numbness of the face, arms, or legs. It could also be difficulty with speaking and trouble understanding what is being said.

Tom's primary symptom was weakness to his legs to the point that he fell. He then had difficulty with speech and understanding so his boss took him directly to the hospital.

Wednesday, August 10, 2005

I feel in a state of limbo. It is like a passage between two things. I am lost between two destinations. My cancer treatment was a fearful journey. I remember wondering if my cancer could be defeated. I wondered if I would have a cure. It is almost one year since my diagnosis. I feel I never had the opportunity to celebrate my cure. So many survivors reflect their joy and happiness. They tell of a new lease on life.

Before I could even comprehend the fact that we won the battle of my cancer, we started a new one – Tom's cancer. My cancer had the word "cure" attached to it. Tom's has the word "terminal" attached to his. I would like to say, how unfair and I have said this. Who is to judge fair and unfair?

Excessively many things have changed this past year. Cancer treatment was the greatest and most demanding and emotional challenge I have ever faced.

Our whole situation makes me cry. I feel depressed, partially since I suppressed the joy I should have been allowed to feel, but felt too guilty to let it happen, and my guilt that Tom has terminal cancer.

My opportunity for celebration became replaced with sadness, pain, worry and sense of being cheated, because Tom now has cancer.

He is a good man. He stood by me, cared for me and worried for me. He loved me during our journey through my cancer, together.

We had no time in between. Boom! We started the radiation, chemo, doctors, hospitals, fatigue, worry and tears before we even had time to dry our tears from my cancer.

Thursday, August 11, 2005

I feel as though I have put my life on hold. I cannot perceive my future. Will it be with or without Tom? I know he is going to die. Dr. H. gave him 9 – 12 months, as of February 2005. November will be nine months. The brain tumors are shrinking, and the lung and adrenal gland tumors are the same as they were in early July with no change to the tumors in his liver. What does that mean? What should I do? Should I live for Tom? Should I do whatever he wants? I have no ideas how to plan a life without Tom, since my life plans have always included him. I realize that I do not have dreams or plans that are just my own.

Tom is my best friend. I rarely do anything that does not include him. How do I begin? Now? After he is gone? Tough questions and I have no answers.

Friday, August 12, 2005

Today ended up being a very emotional day. Tom decided to tell me some of his concerns if he were to die.

He said, "Who will cut the grass after I'm gone?" He was

crying. I guess what he was really saying was, "Who will take care of Rita and my family after I am gone?"

Sunday, August 14, 2005

Tom has gone through a major physical change, especially his face. He is taking medication to reduce the swelling in his brain. The result is that his face is very puffy looking. His hair is gone, and he does not look anything like himself.

We decided to go to the car show in Hammond. As we were walking around, we ran into people we knew. Tom would say hi and they would just stare. When he identified himself and explained the situation, all they would say was "Oh, ok, Good luck" and walk away.

I wonder if people just do not know how to deal with cancer patients. I wonder if it makes people think of their own mortality that makes them so uncomfortable to be around people with cancer. If they only realized, that if they were ever a friend, now would have been the time to show it. Tom became discouraged and wanted to go home.

Monday, August 15, 2005

Tom went to work today and had a CT on his way home. We will get the results in a few days.

Thursday, August 18, 2005

Tom had an appointment with Dr. H. today. Tom is having difficulty breathing resulting from a collapse of his left lung.

Cystourethroscopy - Rita
Monday, August 22, 2005

I had a Cystourethroscopy today. A Cystourethroscopy enables your doctor to see inside your bladder with an endoscope (a tube with a small camera use to perform the test or to do surgery). The doctor found no abnormalities and no explanation for my urinary problems. I was losing faith in this doctor as well.

Friday August 26, 2005

At Tom's appointment, Dr. H. said he suspected that the cancer had moved to Tom's esophagus. He wanted Tom to go for a biopsy on Friday, September 2. It was just before a holiday and the girl's birthday. I guess when it rains, it pours. Actually, it is "When it pours, it reigns". That was the slogan for Morton Salt.

I do not know how to digest this information. If the cancer has spread, I fear Tom's time is greatly reduced. With each passing day, I feel more overwhelmed. It is not just the cancer things, but life now and in the future.

Our plates are so full. Tom is still trying to struggle with going to work. He is struggling to survive chemotherapy. I know he worries about how I will survive after he is gone.

My worries and concerns are pretty much the same as Tom's are. I try to hide my pain and discomforts from him because he does not need to worry about me as well.

I want life to be simple. Other people, family and friends want too much from me at this point in my life. It is not like it used to be, when I had the time and energy, to offer help in any way I could. Now, it overwhelms me, and it seems no one realizes this.

Sometimes it is as though Tom is like a little child. He does want more from me than he ever has. His desire to do things has diminished. He gets confused and is forgetful.

I know he wants to live. Of course, he wants to live. I want him to live also. I guess I have given up hope that he will live. So many things are against him. I sense that some days he realizes that he is going to die, but still does not want to talk too much about it. I think he feels that if he accepts that he is going to die, he will become discouraged. I guess denial right now is his sense of hope.

Monday, August 29, 2005

I started a web page on Caring Bridge so I could keep everyone informed of Tom and my progress without having to repeat it all the time.

Tuesday, August 30, 2005

Lately my main emotional frame of mind is frustration. Tom's hearing loss is frustrating for both of us and so is his memory loss. His comprehension is poor, but I am not sure if he is aware of this.

Tom's mood swings range from irritation, anger, and frustration. I have been trying so hard to do things to make him happy. I work on the house, canning, and internet selling. Whatever it is, he wants me to do, and I try to do it. I am so unsure of what I am supposed to be doing to make his life better without making mine worse.

Another frustration I am dealing with is my fatigue. I presently have a respiratory infection and am on antibiotic. It is really taking its toll on my energy and concentration.

Thursday, September 1, 2005

I am continuing my anti-depressant.

Tom's Second Lung Biopsy
Friday, September 2, 2005

Phillip and I took Tom to St Paul for his second lung biopsy. Once again, Lindalee and Jeff came for support. Even though the test indicated that the cancer had not moved to his esophagus, it did indicate that he had blockage in his left lung. There is an 80% collapse of the lung in the lower lobe and a 50% collapse of the lung on the left upper lobe. Therefore Tom was having so much difficulty breathing.

It was obvious that the cancer was progressing to its life-threatening phase.

It became obvious that Tom's next chemotherapy would not be able to wait until November or December like Dr. H. had hoped.

Saturday, September 3, 2005

Tom has been upset since yesterday with his test results. He told me that he wanted the doctor to "just cut it out of me". I feel helpless with no answers to give him comfort. I just told him that he must keep hoping that something will come along that may extend his life or even offer a cure. It is always possible.

Knowing that someone you love is going to die just eats away at you every day.

Tuesday, September 6, 2005

It is difficult to plan my life after Tom. He insists he is going to be here two years from now. With the re-growth of his tumor, I do not think he will be. I hope that I am wrong. His health seems to be deteriorating more lately and his fight has become increasingly difficult for him.

Wednesday, September 7, 2005

Each day I can feel my faith and hope in Tom's cure fading away. I feel like a traitor to Tom by losing my faith. I feel guilty if I do not have faith in his survival. It is as if I am simply accepting his dying almost like I no longer care to fight anymore.

I went from fighting my cancer into fighting Tom's canner. He went from fighting mine to fighting his. We are both tired.

Thursday, September 8, 2005

One year ago, today, I started my radiation and chemotherapy. Six months ago, I wouldn't have believed that I would ever feel like a human being again.

Tom and I had appointments with Dr. H. today. My skin is healing well and there is no sign of recurrence of my tumor.

The appointment continues with Dr. H. discussing Tom's future chemotherapy. There is no new growth in the esophagus, but the lung tumor has increased in size. His blood counts were high enough so it he would start chemotherapy again tomorrow. Since Tom's ears were still bothering him, another appointment to see the ear specialist was also set up.

It is very rough. I remember being extremely sick and wanting to quit treatment.

I need to renew hope for Tom. He starts chemo again tomorrow. I really hate writing chemotherapy on the calendar again. I guess it is best to take it one day at a time. I need to pretend he is going to live and maybe that will be my hope.

I keep getting repeated bladder infections and less urine control as time passes. Dr. H. suspects that my problems may be related to radiation damage from my treatments. I will need to have further discussions about this with Dr. B.

Cycle Seven – Chemotherapy
Friday, September 9, 2005

Tom has a lot of guts and determination. His tenacity is so great, and it is easy to see that he is strong willed and a fighter.

This cycle of chemotherapy is cycle seven and the first session. It will be for five hours, once every three weeks. The nurse had some difficulty getting the IV into Tom's vein today.

Chemotherapy continues to be hard on Tom's veins. The veins begin to weaken and can collapse or become sensitive to needles making them seem to roll to hide from the needle. The rolling of veins is a physical response of the body to repeated needle pricks. It is not a conscious response. The veins may also become hard, making it more difficult to insert an IV.

She suggested that maybe he should get a port.

IV Port

An IV Port or Portacath administers chemotherapy drugs into the veins instead of an IV insertion into a blood vein. Again, Tom said he was not interested at this time.

Tom is not as interested in watching videos as he had been. He mostly sleeps during treatment. I read or work on some beadwork. I feel supportive and try to encourage him by sitting with him during treatments. He has told me many times that I did not need to come with him during treatments. I told him I wanted to be there. I have seen so many people sit for hours during treatment with no one to talk to and no one giving them support. I do not want to do that to Tom.

Tom seemed to handle his chemo well today. He did not get nauseous or have any stomach problems. He is tired but still goes to work.

Tuesday, September 13, 2005

It is getting more and more difficult to get along peacefully with Tom. He becomes angry or frustrated so quickly and seemingly for no reason. He grumbles and complains a lot, about nothing at all.

This is a total change for him. He has always been emotionally stable and looked at things rationally. After all, he is an engineer. He looks at problems and projects and comes up with applications and solutions.

I become angry because his anger is aimed at me. It may be about the kids, house, or some other reason I have no control over, but it is aimed at me. I know it is the cancer progressing throughout his brain, that is causing such a personality change, but it is still hard for me to adjust.

I am tired and physically worn out. My patience is thin, and I cannot shake the feelings of depression that keep creeping in.

Among Tom's many personally changes are that of being paranoid. He checks on me all the time lately. He wants to know what I am doing at all times. He used to call me once a day from work just before he was leaving. These daily calls were to ask me if I needed anything from town. I loved those calls.

Now he is calling me several times during the day just to see what I am doing. Tom has never worried about where I was or what I was doing. We had always given each other our space so it seems strange to have him "checkup" on me.

Thursday, September 15, 2005

Tom had an appointment with the hearing specialist again today. He has a 50% hearing loss. The doctor had considered putting tubes in his ears but decided against it. The doctor made an incision into the left ear and there was no fluid buildup, so he did not need tubes. The same thing happened to the right ear. Tom will go back in a few weeks and see if hearing aids might help.

To help me remember that Tom's anger is not directed at me personally, I am wearing a porcupine quill bracelet with leather straps hanging down. There are beads on the end of the straps. When they touch against my wrist, it reminds me to be kind to Tom, even if he is seemingly mean to me. It is a gentle reminder, but already it seems to help.

Tuesday, September 20, 2005

I am frustrated with the world. I wish everyone would leave me alone for a while. Other people continue with their lives as though my life were normal, just because their lives are.

I wish people could understand that I am not the same person I was before my cancer treatments. I no longer have the energy to be involved in community activities, a social get together or projects they may have in mind for me.

Wednesday, September 21, 2005

I am sitting in the doctor's office for my appointment. Seeing doctors is getting incredibly old. I am still in my leave me alone mood.

Dealing with Tom is all the stress I can handle. I have not decided if the stress is more me than Tom.

I do not want to talk with anyone. You know that chit-chat stuff. Nobody wants to hear my woes and I guess I am tired of talking about it. However, if I do not talk about it, it bottles up and I become more stressed.

I am becoming more frustrated with having to wear protective under garments all the time. I cringed when I hear all the jokes about it. I am frustrated with wetting my pants and the bed. I am frustrated with the lack of bowel control. I am having a difficult time adjusting to these changes in my lifestyle.

I also cannot seem to organize my thoughts. It seems like my thoughts race all over the place all the time. Concentration is difficult. I cannot relax and I cannot sleep. I feel sad most of the time.

Monday, September 26, 2005

I had an anal ultrasound today. The good news is that I am still tumor and cancer free. The bad news is that there is permanent damage to the sphincter muscle. This cannot be repaired because the surrounding tissue is damaged from the radiation, and I would not heal from such a surgery.

My Lymph percentage is lower than normal. The damage to my groin lymph from radiation treatments are contributing to the lower count.

Wednesday, September 27, 2006

Tom went to the doctor today because of foot pain. Tom had dealt with gout in his foot before, so it was a possibility this was the reason for his most recent pain.

His doctor prescribed Zestril for Tom's hypertension. He also gave him Indocin to help relieve the pain and inflammation.

I am continuing to have both bladder and bowel problems. The results from my cystoscopy indicated that there were no cysts or tumors present in my bladder. This is good news.

Tom's hair is falling out again. I miss the little go-T he had for a while. He is still working.

Friday, September 30, 2005 - Chemotherapy

Today was the second session of cycle seven of Tom's chemotherapy. Tom's veins are doing better these days. Possibly, because his treatments are further apart. What little hair Tom grew back, is now falling out.

Tuesday, October 4, 2005

I am still in my leave me alone me. A part of me is starting to believe that Tom is going to survive for couple of years, rather than months. He is starting to do so well, and I think that is a big part of survival. He is still working, which is impressive. Of course, my thinking may just be wishful.

Just when I think I am gaining a positive outlook; I find myself slipping back into sadness. I started psychological counseling at locally. I am not sure what to expect from this. I need to learn to love life, forgive myself, and stop being judgmental. I also need to develop an interest in life.

Sunday, October 9, 2005

My uncle Jack Miller died on Thursday. He lived in Gordon when Tom was growing up. He is also a Vietnam veteran. It was his injuries in Vietnam in 1972, which finally cost him his life on October 5, 2005.

Tom and I drove up separately for Jack's memorial service. Jack and Tom shared many of the same friends. Tom visited with them at the memorial. Many of them did not know that Tom had cancer.

I remained in Danbury for the funeral the next day and

143

Tom drove the hour and a half home alone. After he left, I felt guilty that I was not with him, but he expressed that he wanted to go to work the next day. I wanted to offer support to my family at the funeral at the loss of Jack.

Monday, October 10, 2005

After speaking to Tom this morning, he told me, he was not going to work. He was too tired.

Thursday, October 13, 2005

Just when I think I am gaining a positive outlook; I find myself slipping back into sadness. I had a severe migraine yesterday. I could not get out of bed and was vomiting quite a bit.

Tom's older brother, Al, is having a major struggle with his alcohol abuse. On Saturday, Tom and I are going to go over and see what we can do to help. We suspect that we will have to bring his dogs to our house for care if he ends up in rehab again. We have gotten him into rehab several times over the past years. I hope one of these times he can find a way to cope with life and remain sober.

Saturday, October 15, 2005

Tom and I went to St Paul to his brother's house. When we arrived, I was not surprised at what I saw. When his brother has a drinking binge, he neglects his house, his eating, and his health. The only thing he does not neglect, even when drinking heavily, is his dogs. It is interesting that he cares so much about them, that his drinking does not get in the way of their care.

A friend of his, who is also in AA with Al, met us at the house. Tom was feeling tired and the emotional toll of seeing his brother in the state he was in was hard on him.

We ended up taking his bother to hospital rehabilitation with the hopes that this treatment will be helpful.

In turn, Tom and I ended taking his four huskies and their houses home with us.

Monday, October 17, 2005

I am worried about Tom. He seemed to be doing better, reduced cough and a fair energy level. This past week, his cough came back and increased. He is very tired this morning and seems depressed. He has his CT today to see if the new chemo is working. Up until this weekend, I had some hope that he would be around a lot longer than the doctor had given him.

After this weekend, I am not so sure. If I believed that he was going to survive, life seems easier to handle. Now, I am feeling the pressure of sorrow knocking at our door. I am beginning to feel depressed again. Life seems lonely and black if I think Tom will not survive.

The weekend dealing with his brother and the dogs took a lot out of Tom. I think he is wondering what will happen to his brother if he were to die. Over the years, Tom has been Al's main support person. Tom feels a responsibly for his brother and I am sure he is worried about what will happen to Al in the future if he is not there to help him.

Tuesday, October 18, 2005

I had my first mental health therapy session with a counselor today. I am not sure where these sessions will take me, but I feel better knowing I am trying to get my thoughts and feelings in order.

Thursday, October 20, 2005 - Chemotherapy

Tom had his seventh cycle – third session today. The chemotherapy continues to beat up on his body. He is very tired and can't seem to shake his depression. I have run out of ideas on how to cheer him up. I guess it is not really cheer him up; it is more like to comfort him. I have no idea what I can do to accomplish comfort for him.

Monday, October 24, 2005

The chemo on Thursday went well for Tom. He did experience some stomach pain, but only for a short while. He is tired this morning. It is amazing how all the doctors, hospitals and treatments start to wear on you. Tom and I have been at this for fourteen months between the two of us.

My counselor said to live one day at a time and to make the best of each day. She also said not to worry about the uncertainties of the future. I could die before Tom.

That, to me, would be tragic for Tom. He would never

survive without me. I am important to his survival. As things go, I am grateful I did survive my cancer so I can be here for Tom. If his having cancer was a part of his fate, whether I survived or not, I am grateful to be here to help him through his struggles.

Tuesday, October 25, 2005

Tom and I both went to the clinic today to get our Flu and Pneumonia shots.

Thursday, October 27, 2005

I went to the doctor today because my headaches did not improve. She will continue me on the Cymbalta for depression. She wants to set me up for an MRI/MRA of the brain and MRI of cervical spine. I guess she wants to see if anything bad is going on in my brain.

Of course, this makes me panic. What if a new cancer has developed in my brain? I am not going to discuss this with Tom. He has enough to worries of his own. I think that as a cancer survivor, I am still fearful it may return.

I had an appointment with my counselor too. We continued to discuss my present situation. We discussed my discomfort about wearing protective under garments. I told her that it bothered me because it was uncomfortable, and I felt stereotyped. She suggested that I design an under garment that would be more comfortable and fashionable for women my age.

I guess that is what bothered me so much about it. Protective undergarments are stereo typed for other women. At 52 years old, I do not consider myself as an "older" woman, not yet.

Thursday October 28, 2005

I was having some suicidal thoughts and discussed this with my personal doctor today. My doctor changed my antidepressant to Cymbalta. Since my blood pressure was running on the low side, she also discontinued the blood pressure medications as well.

Friday, October 28, 2005

Tom got a Procrit shot today. The shot is to help increase red blood cells. Any time Tom's red blood cells are too low; he will not receive his chemotherapy.

Saturday, October 29, 2005

I had a brain and neck MRI today. I know I am having neck problems again maybe because I am more active. It could have to do with stress also. I pray I do not have any brain problems or tumors.

Monday, October 31, 2005

Last year at this time, I had just finished my cancer treatments. Sandy was still here. I miss her a lot. I remember feeling so lousy and fatigued. This year I feel better, but not as good as I used to feel, but better. I am still having leg and hip pain. I hope that improves.

Tom is tired these days and getting more leg and foot pain.

He is excited, however, because we are going to Las Vegas this Sunday. We are staying until Thursday. The anticipation of the trip is making him happy.

Thursday, November 3, 2005

Tom has an upper respiratory infection and is again on antibiotic. He is also suffering from anemia (lack of health red blood cells) and has a mild sore throat. I hope that he will feel well enough to go to Las Vegas next week. He is looking forward to it. He is on Vicodin for the muscle pain he is experiencing, which may be a result of the Taxol chemotherapy drug.

I am continuing my counseling sessions. The sessions give me things to think about, but I am not sure if this is enough.

Saturday, November 5, 2005

Tom is breathing much better and said he feels up to going to Las Vegas, so our plans are still set to go.

Sunday, November 6, 2005

We went to airport for our flight to Las Vegas today. It was a lot of work for me to handle the entire luggage. Tom was feeling tired, and I did not want to wear him out before we even started our mini vacation.

Tom had a handicapped seat, so he had room for his legs. We also brought a personal blanket for him because he has been getting cold. It seems he is cold most of the time now.

My seat was supposed to be across from his but was a row back. It worked out ok. I guess I am so worried that he is going to collapse at any time that I do not want to be to far from him.

I did experience leg and hip pain and discomfort on the flight. That relates back to the destroyed lymph nodes on my groin area. I was grateful to get off the plane so I could relieve some of the leg pain. We had a car rental ready for us when we arrived and went straight to the hotel.

Monday, November 7, 2005

Tom wanted to see other casinos while we were there. He had enough energy to walk to nearby casinos but was exhausted by the time we got to the one across the street. I got a wheelchair for Tom to use at each casino we stopped at.

I was surprised at how difficult and exhausting it was for me to push him around. Most of the pain seemed to be in my hips. We managed and Tom had a great time. He does enjoy gambling.

Tuesday, November 8, 2005

Tom was so tired, that he slept most of the day. His brother Dave had offered to pay for a helicopter tour of the Grand Canyon, but Tom was so exhausted that he decided not to go.

We forgot his medication for the pain in his foot. I did manage to get the prescription sent to the local Wal-Mart and picked it up for him. Once the pain subsided in his foot, he did manage to enjoy a little gaming before bed.

Wednesday, November 9, 2005

We drove to Hoover Dam today. It was long ride, but I did all the driving. We enjoyed ourselves there, but Tom slept once we got back to the hotel.

I found myself spending most of my time alone. I would bring food to the room for Tom and after he ate, he would go back to sleep. I spent my time in the casino alone.

Tom and I ate a light breakfast and spent about an hour playing some of the machines before we went to the airport. He was not feeling much better. Once we got home, he went to sleep.

Friday, November 11, 2005

When we went into the hospital the next morning for Tom's chemo treatment, he did not receive it. His blood work indicated that his white count was dangerously low. Instead of chemo, he received a blood transfusion. He received two units of blood. His hemoglobin was only 6.4, his white count only 1,000 and his platelets were only 30. All of them dangerously low.

I got the results from my MRI. The MRI showed foci in some parts of my brain. These are common with patients who have a history of migraines, of which I have. The MRI did not show any growths or tumors. This is incredibly good news.

Saturday, November 12, 2005

It is becoming more and more difficult to watch the changes in Tom. Life is slowly leaving him, and I cannot do anything to stop it. I realize that the one-year survival is not to mark surviving the cancer but surviving the treatments. The human body can only take just so much chemo and then give up.

I think after this next round of chemo will be all Tom will be able to take for a while. If the tumors become smaller, it may give Tom four to six months before the next round of chemo.

Thursday, November 17, 2005

Tom had a series of CT today, which included chest, abdomen, and pelvis. Tom is breathing better, and his lung collapse has improved. His blood cells are higher, but still low.

We had cake and ice cream for Phillip's birthday.

Monday, November 21, 2005

I went to the doctor today because my urination problem was getting worse, and I felt as though I may have a bladder infection. The doctor put me on Cipro for ten days for a urinary tract infection (UTI).

Monday, November 28, 2005

Tom's blood cells are higher but still too low for chemotherapy.

Tuesday, December 6, 2005

Tom and I both had lab and CT exams today. We will get

the result at our next appointments with Dr. H.

Thursday, December 8, 2005

Tom and I had appointments with Dr. H. today.

Tom's recent CT indicated that the lung tumor was responding to chemotherapy, but there was an increase in the number of tumors in his brain. Dr. H. had stopped Tom's chemotherapy for a while because his blood counts were too low. Tom's concentration is becoming more difficult for him. Even simple tasks cause him frustration. The blood supply to Tom's brain is restricted due to damage to the blood vessels. There were some indications that there may be a possibility of bone metastases.

He does not complain about his lack of hearing anymore and never mentions the ringing in his ears. He is doing the best he can.

Dr. H. discussed using an oral chemotherapy drug called Temodar starting in January. We had discussed Stereotactic Radiosurgery or Gamma-knife surgery for the tumors in his brain, but Tom has too many to lesions to consider this procedure.

Stereotactic Radiosurgery – Gamma-Knife Surgery

Stereotactic Radiosurgery (SRS) treats brain disorders with a focused and precise, single, high dose of radiation. It is usually a single day procedure. It is generally affective on one or two tumors.

Gamma-Knife Surgery is a non-invasive (not penetrating the body, as by incision or injection) when traditional brain surgery is not an option. Contrary to its name, a knife is not used. Instead, the procedure uses powerful doses of radiation to target and treat diseased brain tissue while leaving surrounding tissue intact.

Friday December 9, 2005

Tom's blood counts are still too low for him to have chemo again currently. His red count is only 7.5 and his platelets are very low. If the count does not increase by the end of the week, he will have to have another blood transfusion.

Saturday, December 10, 2005

I finally got all the items together to apply for my Social Security disability for myself. I hope I am eligible with my bladder and bowel problems. I am so insecure about going into public and having an accident with either. I have to go to the bathroom every half hour to forty-five minutes and have no warning about my bowels. Combined with my neck, spine, and hip problems I hope I am eligible.

I have been working on it for the past few months. If I am on my own, I may have to live on Social Security Disability. I hate to think about these things, but they will be part of my future if Tom is gone.

Tuesday, December 13, 2005

Tom had lab and CT today and I had lab. Even though Tom's blood counts are still low, they are increasing each day. They are still too low for chemotherapy.

His CT showed that Tom has damage to the central nervous system due to the number of lesions in the white matter of the brain. He also has some infection of the mastoid bone of the skull, which is located behind the ear. This is possibly from the repeated ear infections he gets.

Wednesday, December 14, 2005

Tom has a non-productive cough and has increasing confusion. Tom was going to work this morning and decide to take the Tahoe. While he was leaving, he backed into the side of the Del Sol. The whole door caved in and crunched the front fender. Since Tom hit one of our cars with another of our cars, insurance will not cover it. This is yet another disappointment in our lives. The Del Sol is Tom's baby and neither he nor I are in good enough health to fix it. It will have to wait. I think it has become time for me to drive Tom back and forth to work. Driving is becoming more difficult for him lately.

He decided he would give up driving for a while. I will now give him a ride back and forth to work each day and take him to all his appointments.

Tom has been showing signs of Cushingoid features and

these symptoms have worsened. His face is very puffy and round looking.

Cushingoid

Cushingoid is a term used in medicine to suggest that a person has symptoms or appearance similar to what would be expected if that person were suffering from Cushing's disease. Cushing's disease is a condition affecting the pituitary gland where the body overproduces cortisol.

Cushingoid facial features are characteristic of a round, puffy and moon-faced appearance.

Friday, December 16, 2005

Sandy and Larry are here from Oregon again because his mother, Dora is not doing very well. Her doctors told them she might not survive more than a week or two.

Saturday, December 17, 2005

Tom and I went to the cities to visit with Dora. It was sad to see her so lifeless. She has always been so positive about life. It was evident that she would not make it much longer.

Tom and I got home and got ready for his company Christmas party.

It was very surreal for us to be at the party with Tom now a cancer patient. Last year I was the cancer patient. Tom did not want to stay long as he was tired. We, however, managed to dance one slow dance before we left.

Sunday, December 25, 2005

We spent Christmas in Gordon. The Christmas dinner and get together was celebrated at Mary's house, Tom's mother. The gathering was so unique this year because not only were there members of Tom's family present but some of my family members as well. My parents, our children, and Sandy and Larry joined us.

We played a fun dice pass around game where a pair on the die earned you a gift. A particular set of carved wooden fish on a stringer caught Tom's eye. He tried very hard to keep it, but it kept eluding him. When the game was ended, Larry was in possession of the wooden fish. He walked over to Tom and gave them to him. Tom's faced just beamed.

I will cherish this special and memorable Christmas for a long time.

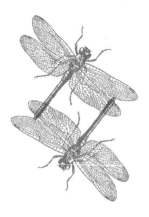

CHAPTER 11 - HOPE FADES

DXA Exam (Dual Energy X-ray Absorptiometry)
Tuesday, December 27, 2005

Today I had a DXA exam, also called DEXA scan or bone densitometry exam. This test is used to measure the mineral density in bone. During the exam, two x-rays with different levels of energy are aimed at the area of concern, and the absorption rate of the x-rays is used to calculate the concentration of minerals like calcium in the bones.

The test was painless. The machine sends an invisible beam through the bones being examined. The areas most tested are the spine and hip areas. During the exam, I lay on a table and the machine passed over my waist and hips. It was quite simple and very quick. I will get the test results in about a week.

Winter Road Trip
Wednesday, December 28, 2005

Larry had to return to work, but Sandy decided to stay an additional week.

Sandy, Tom, and I decided to go to Hinckley, MN to the local casino, but accidently made reservations for the sister casino near Onamia, MN instead. It was one hundred miles further away. We decide to "just go" and see where it took us. We wanted an adventure.

We had fun at the casino and slept very well that night. The next morning, to our surprise, it had snowed several inches. We never thought to check the weather forecast before we left home. The hotel had no openings for the night, so we were forced to hit the road. The next closet place to stay was the casino we originally wanted. It was only sixty miles away, but with all that snow it seemed like a thousand miles. I was grateful to have our four-wheel drive. I only recently took over all the driving and winter driving has always been my nemesis.

The roads were icy and unplowed. I had white knuckles the entire drive. There were cars and semi-trailers in the ditch all along our route. When we finally got to the hotel, I was extremely relieved and could not wait to get into our room.

I will not soon forget this adventure.

Friday, December 30, 2005

We laughed all the way home from the second casino as we recalled how foolish we had been in not checking the weather. It felt good to do something spontaneous.

Sunday, New Year's Eve 2006

Since Tom was not feeling up to cooking, the duty of making our traditional lobster New Year's Eve dinner fell upon me. I have never cooked a live lobster in my entire life. I was not looking forward to it. Tom laughed when I was reluctant to drop the poor lobster in the boiling water. It is not as easy as it sounds, but I managed to serve a nice dinner after all.

Tuesday, January 2, 2006

Sandy went home today. It was enjoyable to have her here for a visit.

Thursday, January 4, 2006

Tom had an appointment with Dr. H. today. The tumors in his brain have multiplied and increased in size. The tumors in his lung and adrenal glands have decreased.

Tom has not had chemotherapy since November because his blood counts have not increased enough for him to be able to handle it. Dr. H. is starting Tom on an oral chemotherapy drug that will potentially affect the brain tumors.

Tom is changing a lot. Physically, he is like a seventy-year-old man. His shoulders are hunched over; he is pale and losing his balance.

Mentally, he is like a ten-year-old child.

His concentration is worse than ever. He has to think several minutes about what he is doing before he can accomplish it.

He is being very accusing to me. He tells me I am not being supportive. I know I am doing everything he wants me to do and the things I need to do. I realize these comments are coming from the damage the tumors are doing to his brain. His personality change has been occurring slowly over the past few months.

It hurts me to see him deteriorate like this. The man I love and knew is slowly slipping away every day. I feel helpless because I cannot do anything to stop it.

Cycle One - Oral Chemotherapy – Temodar
Brain Blood Membrane
Thursday, January 5, 2006

Tom started the first cycle of oral chemotherapy today, called Temodar (temozolomide – generic). This drug crosses the blood membrane of the brain, and it is hoped to have a positive effect on the brain tumors. The blood membrane is a barrier that restricts the passage of substances, such as chemotherapy, to protect the brain from damage.

The brain has a protective membrane that does not allow traditional IV chemotherapy drugs to cross over to the brain, but an oral drug has more potential to affect the tumors.

An oral chemotherapy drug is absorbed by the stomach, which allows it to pass through the blood membrane to the brain. Not all chemotherapy drugs can be delivered this way due to the toxicity of the drug. Either the stomach cannot absorb many chemotherapy drugs, or they are too toxic for the stomach to handle.

Tom's cycle will consist of five days of one dose each day and repeated twenty-three days later. He could experience similar side effects from an oral chemotherapy as those he experienced form the IV delivered drugs. We had detailed instructions on storage and handling.

Friday, January 6, 2006

Today is the second day of Tom's cycle one of oral chemotherapy. I do hope this new chemo treatment is beneficial to Tom's survival.

I have been racking my brain to find ways to deal with the behavior changes that Tom is exhibiting. He has begun to lie about simple things. He puts me down in his conversations. He has not quit smoking and is trying to hide it from me. He hides cigarettes and is hoarding cigarette lighters.

He has become more demanding, erratic, and angry. His physical changes continue. His vision is becoming worse, his ability to taste has demised and his memory has not improved. He is now experiencing muscle and leg weakness and loss of balance. I continue to drive him back and forth to work. He admitted that his concentration is not good enough for him to be driving at all.

Saturday, January 7, 2006

Today is the third day of Tom's cycle one of oral chemotherapy. He does not express how he feels emotionally about this process. I can imagine his thoughts are full of hope that this drug will reduce the brain tumors.

Sunday, January 8, 2006

As cycle one, day four begins, Tom seems to be having some nausea for the Temodar. Reluctantly he is now taking Compazine to help control it but is unhappy with the drossiness it causes.

Rachel and Valerie came home to visit their dad today. When Tom was taking a nap, the girls said they wanted to have a discussion with me.

They asked me if I thought it would be a good idea if they deferred their college by a semester.

"We could be around to help out with dad more and spend time with him." Rachel explained.

I was touched by their thoughtfulness.

"Right now," I explained, "One of the most important things to your dad is that you both graduate college. He may live long enough to see you graduate if you finish off your last semester now."

"One of the greatest gifts you can give to your dad is the knowledge that you will be graduating in May. It is very important to him. It is his legacy."

The girls both agreed and decided that they would finish the year so their dad could see them graduate in May.

Monday, January 9, 2006

I am happy today is the fifth and last day of cycle one of the oral chemotherapy. The drug has made Tom increasingly tired since he started taking it. I hope the Temodar can help to decrease the brain tumors. There does not seem to be any other treatment currently.

Tuesday, January 10, 2006

It is becoming more complicated to keep track of my and Tom's appointments, and Tom's chemotherapy, both oral and IV. In order to keep things straight, I designed a calendar to mark all appointments, chemotherapy, vitamins and nutrition. I hope this chart/calendar will make things easier for both of us.

Post Radiation Osteoporosis – Rita
Wednesday, January 11, 2006

Just when I think I cannot handle any more negative information; it comes my way. The results of my DXA text indicated that I have severe osteoporosis.

Radiation to the pelvic area results in demineralization of bone matrix, increasing the risk of osteoporosis and pelvic fractures. These risks increase with age especially women over 60 years old. Women treated with pelvic radiation for anal cancer have the highest risk of pelvic fractures.

Osteoporosis is a possible permanent side effect that I was

not aware of at the time of my treatment. Since I did not have a DXA prior to radiation, I have no way of knowing if I had this condition already. I did not have the hip and leg pain I have now, so it is hard to determine.

At 50 years old at the time of my treatments and I should not have been considered a high risk. I will have to learn to deal with it the best that I can.

Thursday, January 12, 2006

Dr. H. expressed that he felt Tom was handling the oral Temodar quite well and he would continue with his present schedule. He did say he would not continue the IV chemotherapy at this time.

Friday, January 13, 2006

I went to the spine specialist today for an evaluation of my recent neck pain. I have been to this doctor several times in the past years. I have been dealing with degenerative spine and nerve damage in both my upper and lower spine.

He recommended that I receive an epidural at C5-6. I had good results with it the last time I had it done. He also recommended physical therapy, but I already know that it is not going to be possible. With everything that is happening with Tom right now, I just cannot plan on that.

Saturday and Sunday, January 14 - 15, 2006

We spent the weekend at my mom and dad's house. Tom and dad went ice fishing. Tom and my dad had portable fishing shacks that would zipper together to make one large shack.

Since Tom is so cold all the time lately, he brought a portable heater to put inside the shack. His two brothers, Marty and Dave also went fishing. They told us afterwards how humorous it was to stand outside of Tom and dad's shack. Both Tom and dad are hard of hearing so as they were "talking", their very loud voices boomed crossed the frozen lake. I can just imagine how funny it was.

They were proud of their catch, and we took pictures to commemorate the event. After cleaning the fish, we froze them to take home for future eating.

Monday, January 16, 2006

I started Fosamax to help reduce my risk of bone fractures. Fosamax is a bisphosphonate that works to help slow down or reduce bone loss and help to increase the bone density. I take it once a week. I hope is helps with my hip and leg pain, even though I am not certain they are related. I am concerned about the expenses of an adding another prescription. We have so many already between both Tom and me.

The more I analyze our financial future, the more concerned I become. Tom wants a new car. I would love him to have a new car, but if we do not get his company's recent minimal life insurance benefit, and Tom dies, I do not think I can handle both a house and a car payment. We do not have Life and Casualty on the house, which still has a substantial mortgage.

Sunday, January 22, 2006

There are so many thoughts and feelings that I keep to myself. While I am trying to cope with the possibility that Tom may die, I am afraid to share any of these feelings with anyone. I am afraid they will think I have given up on Tom's survival. I have not given up but have become fearful that he will die.

I am trying to convince myself not to feel guilty about moving on after he dies. I know Tom would want me to have a good life, even if he cannot.

Part of me is worried that I will not be able to handle all the changes and meet all his needs as he regresses in the weeks to come. Occasionally, when he does mention his own death, he tells me he wants to die at home. I will fulfill this wish for him no matter how much of a demand it is one me. I love him and I know he would do the same for me.

Tuesday, January 24, 2006

I am finding it more difficult to watch Tom die as the days go by. I wish his body had changed sooner than his mind. If his thinking and comprehension were better than it presently is, we could still communicate our thoughts and feelings with each other. The treatments and the cancer continue to take their toll on him, giving way to a losing battle every day. Reality is weighing heavy on me and I feel helpless. I cannot stop it and I hate accepting it.

Tuesday, January 31, 2006

The transmission went out on the Tahoe today. It needs to be fixed so we can plow the driveway and it is the only vehicle we I have running right now. Larry is arranging for a discount on the transmission and the dealer in town will install it. My sister Val loaned us her car until the Tahoe is fixed.

Cycle Two - Oral chemotherapy
Wednesday, February 1 - 5, 2006

Tom started his second cycle of oral chemotherapy. His is experiencing tiredness but the nausea is under control. He is not saying too much, about how he feels or expressing any hopes or concerns.

Sandy called this weekend and told me about the plans her and Larry were making to move from Oregon back to the Midwest. She said that they wanted to come and help me with Tom. I was touched by her thoughtfulness. She said they would keep me informed about their progress and when they may be able to come back.

Wednesday, February 8, 2006

Today is the one-year anniversary of Tom's diagnosis. It is difficult to put all the things that have happened over the past year into perspective. We are dealing with things as they arise. Tom is getting weaker these days. I am driving him to work each day and picking him up. He does not seem to mind. He does not say anything about it.

Saturday, February 11, 2006

Tom's brother Al is going to enter Alcohol Rehab for a ninety-day program. We are once again going to take care of his dogs. Al talked it over with Phillip since this task will fall solely on him. Phillip agreed. The kennels we had when we raised dogs, were still in place, so it was just a matter of getting the dogs moved over here.

Tuesday, February 14, 2006

Today was a good day. It ended up being a long one though. Tom had an MRI and CT test starting at 7:00 in the morning. The nurse had difficulty trying to get an IV into Tom's arm. After two nurses tried and failed, they finally called Linda from the chemo department to do it. She was successful. Tom's arms and hand are very bruised and sore.

After Tom's appointment, I took him to work and then bought some carnations and three balloons with a cute card. After I picked him up from work, we shared our Valentine cards and gifts. Tom enjoyed his and I enjoyed mine. He gave me a crystal angel holding my birthstone and a polished red stone with the word LOVE etched into it.

I made lobster tail, a great salad and scratch pasta salad that turned out wonderful. I added the Bragg vinegar and aminos. I also made the northern he had caught when he and dad went fishing last December. Phillip ate with us. For dessert, I made a double heart cake with walnuts, chocolate chips and coconut.

Tom did not eat very much but he did eat enough to enjoy his meal.

Thursday, February 16, 2006

Tom and I went shopping today and he cut his finger on a shopping cart. With his platelets so low, Tom bleeds easily from even a small cut. I carry a small first aid kit in my purse with band-aids and gauze. We were standing in the store trying to stop the bleeding. I was surprised how much blood there was. After about five minutes, we got the bleeding stopped.

Sandy and Larry are getting their lives organized for their move back to the Midwest. Sandy said it is time to move back not only to help Tom and I but also to help with our aging parents. Larry also wants to re-connect with his family. They have been gone seventeen years. It is a difficult decision for them to make. The biggest choice was to leave their children and grandchildren. Now that they have decided to leave Oregon, they are preparing for the move.

Friday, February 17, 2006

Tom seems to be doing well but he still losing his balance occasionally.

He is having bouts of aggression lately. He is upset because everybody treats him so differently because he has cancer. He said that they persecute him for it. He says I do too. He tells me I tell him how to live his life and he does not like it. I guess I worry about his health and feel I have ideas to share with him to make it better, but he sees it as me interfering with his life.

It is difficult at times because he does not see things that way. He just sees it as me trying to control him. I just try to encourage him to eat and drink water. However, again he sees it as me controlling him. I am trying to back off. I guess it is his life and if he wants to do things that may shorten his life; I cannot do anything about it. I just try to assure him that I love him and that I want the best for him.

His CT results indicated that the brain tumors have not decreased but they have not increased either. That is good news. Unfortunately, the lung tumor has begun to grow again. He will start the IV chemotherapy again next week. He is still going to work every day. I am amazed by his strength and endurance.

Saturday, February 18, 2006

Tom fell outside on the deck today. I had a difficult time getting him up. This concerns me. What if he falls and gets hurt? I am afraid this is going to happen more often as time goes by. We did get a wheelchair from his mother, so when if we go anywhere that requires a lot of walking, I push him in it.

I feel the pain in my legs and hips when I push him, but I am not going to tell him about the pain.

Cycle Eight – Chemotherapy
Monday, February 20, 2006

Tom started the eight cycle, session one of IV chemotherapy. I am concerned about his endurance. He is receiving two types of chemo and I fear that his body will not be able to handle too much more.

There are times I wish I had a shoulder to cry on. Unless

someone is going through what you are, it is difficult for them to understand. Most of the time when I express my feelings, I am told about all the people who feel they bad deal in life as well. Instead of trying to understand my feelings, they just tell me about other people's feeling expecting me to accept my dilemma as an everyday thing. I do not understand.

I try and not let Tom see how I feel, but we have been at this for over a year with Tom and a year and a half combined. The more worn down I become, the harder and harder it is to hide my feelings. I feel as though no one can imagine how I feel. How could they know unless they were wearing my shoes? How could they even know?

It is at times like this, that I imagine I will not want to live after Tom is gone. I do not see the value in life. With my children grown and moving on with their own lives, I do not want to start all over again.

However, after more thought, I know that my kids will need me more than ever once their dad is gone. Just the thought of living without Tom fills me with fear. It is fear of having to do everything alone and all by myself. The fear of making decisions I am not used to making and the fear of losing my best friend.

Tuesday, February 21, 2006

I feel a lot of anger today at everyone and everything. Life is not supposed to be so sad, so depressing, and so useless. I cannot handle life anymore. I feel so sad that my gut hurts. Tension and pain to the point that my eyes well with tears and all I want to do is cry.

My breathing is strained, and I just want to hide somewhere. I just want it over with, either Tom survives, or he does not. I am tired of doctors, chemo, and all of it. It is not life; it is just an existence and a miserable one at that.

I know Tom is not going to get better, but I must pretend that he is. I have to put up with the anger and the aggression he aims toward me. Each day I want to live less and less.

These thoughts are a shame since Tom is fighting so hard to keep his life. It would be different if I knew he would survive, but I know he will not.

I do not know how he really feels about all of this because he will not talk about it and I do not want to push him. I wish it were easier to accept that he is going to die. I know I will miss him with all my heart and soul. The fear of losing him is messing up my thoughts and I cannot seem to think straight these days.

I hope tomorrow is a better day.

Wednesday, February 22, 2006

I started feeling better today and feel as though I have a sense of direction. I listed a bunch of classic car parts on the internet and a few motorcycle parts. Tom has always enjoyed watching our online auctions and this will give him something to do.

Tom is feeling much better. He still keeps on insisting that I am against him. I guess that is what happens when the brain deteriorates. I hope I have the strength to handle all the things Tom will be going through in the near future.

I feel like going to sleep. I guess I will take a nap and hope I have some energy to get something done when I wake up.

Cycle Three – Oral chemotherapy
Monday, February 27, 2006

The remainder of cycle eight of Tom's IV Chemotherapy is postponed. His blood counts are getting too low. His count cannot handle both the oral and the IV therapies. He is continuing with the oral chemotherapy schedule for now. Today is day one, cycle three of the Temodar.

Wednesday, March 1, 2006

Today was Tom's third does of cycle three of oral chemotherapy. He seems to be tolerating it well. I am sure the oral chemotherapy is contributing to the low blood counts he is having, but we are hopeful this will affect the brains tumors.

I am not sure how I feel today. I can feel the depression creeping in and taking control. When I think of Tom not being here anymore, I do not want to think of my life after him. It does not seem worth it. If Tom knew I had these thoughts, he would be hurt. He is trying so hard to live.

He did not have his IV chemo on Monday because his blood count was too low. That seems to be happening a lot lately. The more of the treatments he misses, the more the potential there is for the tumor to grow. I suspect that deep down he knows he is going to die. I know he had a two-year goal.

I wish I could do something to help make his life complete, but he has not defined what he wishes. I know he has always been financially oriented. If I could get a financial success story in place before his time is up that would bring him peace. I do not want him to know how hard it will be for me once he is gone.

I am waiting to hear about the application for disability for me. Adding the osteoporosis to my list of health conditions may be enough for me to get it. If it does, that will make me unable to work, so my finances will be rough. Nevertheless, I will never share my gloomy financial picture with him. He does not need to know.

Thursday, March 2, 2006

This is day four of cycle three of Tom's oral chemotherapy. There is one more day to go. Our fingers are crossed.

I read in my journal that I had said that I hated my life. I do not hate my life; I hate the things that are happening in it. I am afraid, confused, sad and depressed. The thought of living without Tom leaves me feeling lonely.

I am also afraid of what Tom will go through before the end. I am afraid that I will not be strong enough to support and help him as much as he will need. I will not put him in a nursing home because his wish is to die at home. He deserves that much. Phillip has agreed to help with this when the time comes.

Friday, March 3, 2006

Today is the last day of cycle three of Tom's oral chemotherapy. I am glad that it is over so his body can try to recover. It is sad that he needs two types of chemotherapy in order to have a chance to survive. It is so hard on his body. His tenacity and will to live is so strong, that I wish with all my heart that it were enough. I know it is not.

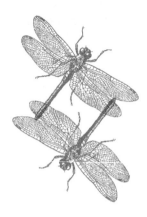

CHAPTER 12 - DEALING WITH TERMINAL

Terminal Illness

A terminal illness is a disease that cannot be cured and is expected to result in death. The timeline may vary from weeks to months and it some cases a limited number of years. The news of being a terminally ill patient is devastating and the first response is generally shock.

Acceptance is difficult for the family but even more so for the patient. Tom has still not accepted that he will die. I wish he would so we could talk about things such as his burial and any last wishes. I get the impression from him that if he accepts that he is going to die then he has given up hope. Hope exists up until the last breath, so accepting the strong possibility of death does not mean all hope is lost. It frees you to address issues that need to be addressed without giving up hope.

Tom has not accepted his emanate death, even though he occasionally mentions that he may die. As his caregiver, I took the responsibility to put into place important issues that need to be addressed. We already took care of two important items, a living will, and an estate will. I know the estate will give Tom peace of mind knowing that I would receive all our assets just in case he did die.

Additional issues that should be taken care of are a Medical Power of Attorney, Hospice care and his burial desires. I do not push these issues with Tom since he believes that I have given up on him if I bring it up. I hope Tom comes to accept his terminal illness before it is too late for him to express any final thoughts.

He is experiencing anticipatory grief and needs to pass through the stages of grief in his own time.

Anticipatory Grief

An aspect of terminal illness is the occurrence of anticipatory grief. This form of grief has many aspects of the grief that loved ones feel after the terminally ill patients dies, only it is experienced by the patient.

Even though Tom has not yet accepted that he is terminal, he is experiencing denial, disbelief, sorrow, and depression. Dying is letting go of future dreams, plans and the people you love. It is also realizing that the people, who love you, must also let go of you.

Loved ones may also experience anticipatory grief, which becomes a different type of grief once their loved one dies.

I have been doing a lot of thinking these past few days. I feel so lost in my life right now. I am so concerned on how to deal with Tom's terminal cancer, and I really wanted some answers. I did some additional research on ideas of how to deal with this time in my life and have found some ideas to consider.

Helping Terminally Ill Patient to Cope

There are many aspects of terminal illness to consider during treatment. These aspects involve feelings, emotions, and unanswered questions.

Tom is changing both physically and mentally. His personality is going through changes as the tumors migrate throughout his brain. He is also experiencing physical function changes such as hearing, sight and motor skills.

We are both at the crossroads of depression, confusion,

stress, and many days of being overwhelmed. Having a guide-line for reference as the disease progresses will be beneficial and serve to remind me how to deal with issues as they arise.

Allow loved one to be in denial: My biggest concern is that Tom has not accepted that he is going to die. I discovered that it is not important for Tom to accept he is dying. Denial is a coping mechanism that is working for him. The reality of his death is frightening to him and overwhelming. Denial is one form of survival that allows us to continue living as we reflect on the possibility of death.

It does seem natural for Tom to respond this way. He is determined and positively stubborn. He has spent his life find-ing solutions to problems. He is trying to find a solution to his present problem, which is to survive his cancer, and is set on a positive outcome. Denial is also way for your loved one to pro-tect the ones they love from the reality of their eminent death.

While Tom is in denial, I know it is important for me to make sure he gets the proper nutrition and medical care. He does get angry with me when he is not hungry and I coax him to eat, or when he does not drink enough water. All I can do is keep trying and do my best.

Help loved one live as normally as possible: When Tom's doctor suggested that Tom stop working and find enjoy-able ways to spend his last days, Tom had no desire to stop working.

Tom has always loved engineering and the unique chal-lenges the field offers. I would tell people that Tom has not worked a day in his life. For him, his job is not work it is ful-fillment. Since Tom has chosen to remain working, I am sup-porting his wishes. I personally would like to see him travel or spend his time in another leisure fashion but working is what he wants.

Be Patient: Doing everyday things are becoming difficult for Tom, but I do not help him until he truly needs it. It may take him longer to accomplish a task, but he receives personal satisfaction in doing it himself. These accomplishments give him a sense of control in a life where he is losing control each passing day.

Be open to communication: I know I get impatient about Tom not addressing his terminal diagnosis. I am afraid that we will not have time to discuss issues that may or may not be important to him to discuss. I avoid forcing him to talk because I know he is not ready. Allow your loved one to share the thoughts and ideas they are ready to share as time goes by.

Tom does not express his emotions easily as most men do not. As a woman, I am more open to expressing my feelings so I must have patience and wait until he is ready.

Be present: One way I show support to Tom is going to his appointments, chemotherapy treatments and tests. Being present sends a message to him that I have not abandoned him. By being available when he feels like talking is another way to show support.

When he is accusing me of giving up on him I continue to assure him, I have not. It is frustrating for me to hear Tom say this, but I realize the progression of his brain tumors cause him to believe I have given up on him.

Offering my insights as a cancer patient is another way, I show my support. I know he values my opinions about side effects and other treatment related issues.

Help with their anticipatory grief: Each terminal patient comes to terms with their future death as different stages of grief. Do not hurry them through their grieving. You want them to live life as fully as possible during their terminal illness. It takes time and each person has his or her own timeline for this process.

Fear of the illness: Possible fears that your loved one may have, is the fear of future pain. I know Tom had some fears about his treatments because he was present during my treatments. He visualized the side effects, pain, and anxieties that I experienced during my treatments. I think this is why he asked Dr. H. if he would get as sick as I had gotten.

Tom is aware of the things to come in the future, as his illness progresses. He will lose control of his bodily functions and fears he will become a burden. When this time comes, it is important to reassure them that they are not a burden. Reinforce that you love them. The feeling of being loved is vital during the end months.

The unknown is fearful, and I know it is fearful for me. Throughout this journey, I need to take care of myself as well. If I do not take care of myself, I cannot take care of Tom.

Helping Yourself Cope

Some thoughts that I have come up with are helpful techniques, some I am using and others I will begin using to help me though this part of our journey.

- **Take control of my life**: I need to continue to live my life and cannot completely revolve it around Tom's illness. I need to be kind and take care of myself and should create a personal quality time. I enjoy beading jewelry or recreational reading, so I will find more time to do these things.

- **Be more aware of my emotions:** I do experience phases of depression and seeing my counselor is a healthy step to deal with these feelings. Spending time talking with my sisters is beneficial as well. With their help, I can talk about things that are bothering me and find a solution for many of those things.

- **Learn how to ask for and accept help from others:** As I was going through my cancer treatments, I learned the importance of asking help from others. I realize that I have not recovered from my cancer treatments and still need to ask for help. Now that I am better, I once again find this difficult. I do; however, realize I cannot do it alone.

Having specific things for people to help with makes it easier for them to decide if they can be helpful or not. Just saying you can help is too vague. Specific tasks will define what I really need help with and give them a defined task. Helping with housework, laundry or grocery shopping are specific things they can be asked to do.

- **Do not forget to live for yourself:** I need to learn not to do everything that Tom wants me to do for him. I will support his independence and let him do as much for himself as possible. I want to make Tom's last days on earth as fulfilling and pleasant as possible, so I was willing to cater to all his wants. The problem with this is that I found myself exhausted and worn out from trying to live both our lives.

- **Trust myself in the decisions I make for Tom:** I need to feel that the decision I make and the ones I encourage Tom to make will be the right ones. In the now and present, I weight the options of his health care, nutrition and activities and make the decisions I feel are the best for him.

- **Allow yourself to grieve**: I am also experiencing anticipatory grief. I am grieving my loss of Tom before he is gone. I need to allow myself to do this, and I am aware that I will start another grieving process after Tom has died. I am to allow myself to move forward and imagine the future in a positive way, even without Tom in my life. I find this very hard to do. I know this one will take a lot more effort for me.

- **Seek out a support group of caregivers:** This type of support will let you know that you are not alone. Through sharing the experiences, thoughts, and feelings of other caregivers, you will learn coping techniques, care helps and emotional support that only other caregivers can offer.

This journey does not have to be traveled alone. Even though exhaustion and stress become your daily companion, seeking advice from others or through reading can help make each day bearable.

Saturday, March 4, 2006

Sandy and Larry are continuing the process of moving

back to Wisconsin. They are making plans for a garage sale and are arranging for a moving van. I talk to Sandy daily on the phone and even though she is far away, her support gives me strength each day. My sister Lindalee also calls me daily and she too gives me encouragement that I can survive this part of my life's journey.

Sunday, March 5, 2006

I do not think God intended for us to suffer so much on our journey through life. I wonder when things went wrong. It changed somewhere. We are told that God is good. That God wants the best for his children. God would not have intended for our lives to be so miserable. I know we need to do all we can to make our lives the best it can be, but so many hurdles get in the way. My thoughts about God and his plans for us are changing. I used to pray but lately I feel praying is a ritual and not an act of faith. Tom's faith is still strong, and I know that his faith is giving him the strength he needs to continue with his fight against his cancer.

Monday, March 6, 2006

Last night I could tell that Tom was having difficulty breathing. I asked him if he was uncomfortable. He replied, "A little".

I asked, "Where are you uncomfortable?"
He did not answer.
I asked, "Is it your legs?"
"A little," he said.
"Is it your lungs?"
"A little."
"Is it as bad as when you had pneumonia?"
"Not that bad," he replied.

Lying in bed last night listening to Tom wheeze has rekindled my sorrow that he will die. Without his chemo treatments, the lung tumors just continue to grow and block his airway. I was hoping he could survive until Rachel and Valerie's graduation from college. Their gradation is his legacy. It is very important to him.

Sorrow is flooding in on me. I was anxious for this to be over, so Tom does not suffer anymore, but now I am not. I do not want Tom to leave. I want him around for a lot longer, even the way he is now. Once he is gone, he is gone. He will not be coming back. That is such an empty feeling. He is so much a part of my life, a part of me. When he is gone, a part of me will go with him.

I know people lose their spouses every day. Sometimes they lose little children.

I am grateful that Tom lived long enough to see his children as responsible and caring adults and they have enjoyed their dad as they grew into adults.

Tom and I have had almost twenty-nine years together. Sometimes were rough, but most times were wonderful. He has been good to me. He made me feel like a member of our team. He did not regulate me and never physically abused me. He is a good man, a good father, and a good husband.

Tuesday, March 7, 2006

Dana Reeves died today from lung cancer after her diagnoses in September 2005. Peter Jennings who was diagnosed in March of 2005, died in July of 2005. I am amazed that Tom is still surviving. He has advanced metastasized small cell lung cancer and is still fighting it fourteen months later.

I do not know why he is still alive. It is his determination, drive and his desire to live. The mind is strong. However, as the tumors take over his brain, the weaker his mind will become. Tom is already becoming less strong. I know he is going to lose his battle. I need to realize this and try to put things into place so Tom can leave this world knowing the rest of us will be fine once he is gone.

Wednesday, March 8, 2006

Tom was up a lot of last night. He was having a lot of leg pain, difficulty breathing and a headache. He seemed better this morning. I am afraid that if he does not get chemo soon, he may not make it to May 13th, the girls graduation day.

Thursday, March 9, 2006

Dr. H. examined me today and said my skin was healing

and looked healthier. He said he saw no indication of any cancer. It was good to hear that. I have enough on my mind as it is. He asked how I was doing, and I broke down crying because I was afraid that Tom would die before the girls' graduation from college.

He told me that Tom was very determined. He said he might make it that long. We would have to wait and see.

Sunday, March 12, 2006

My sister Val, my niece, Christina and her two daughters came over to visit Tom. Tom enjoys having his family near him. I wish his brothers would come and see him, but I guess they have busy lives. I know Al is still in rehab so I understand why he cannot be here.

Monday, March 13, 2006

Tom and I talked a little last night about funeral arrangements. I told Tom I wanted to check into it so we could lock in a low price now, rather than at higher price years from now. I was trying to present it to him in a non-urgent fashion.

He told me he wanted to be cremated, a memorial in Baldwin and buried in Gordon. Pretty much the same as I thought. I felt a sense of relief that we had discussed this issue.

I have been feeling sad the last few days. I do not feel as bitter about our situation as I have. Everybody dies. It happens anywhere from birth to old age. There is no set pattern and no lottery that determines who and when. It just happens. As sad as it is, Dana Reeve spent ten years taking care of her husband, Christopher, watching him strive for improvement and then die.

A year after his death, she was diagnosed with cancer and six months later, she too, died. Their thirteen-year-old son is now alone. How can I complain?

I would like Tom to live longer, but the reality is that he will not. Miracles can happen, but I do not see one happening here. I guess his miracle is that he has survived as long as he has.

He could have died even a year ago if the cancer had not been discovered. That may be our miracle. When I got pneumonia and Tom got it from me, the doctors found his cancer. If it had not happened that way, he could have been dead by April or May of last year.

Miracles are not always what we pray for, and miracles may have already happened; we just do not see them. Sandy was saying that Tom and I had a couple of years of love and renewed romance just before I had my cancer. This too could be a miracle. I have great memories to cherish now that Tom is leaving, rather than be bitter that those times will be gone and will not happen again. I am grateful that we had those times.

Cycle Nine - Chemotherapy
Tuesday, March 14, 2006

Tom's blood count was still good today, so he got his next session of chemo. I have lost track of which drug he is now receiving. I know a certain drug can only be given so many sessions and then has to be changed. The cancer cells develop immunity to the drug after so many treatments and the drug becomes ineffective against the cancer.

Wednesday, March 15, 2006

I must find a way to convince Tom that I will be all right after he is gone. I am not sure what I will do. I am a survivor. I have always been a survivor. I will miss Tom, but I will continue.

Thursday, March 16, 2006

Time is slipping away very quickly. It is almost Tom's birthday again.

This has been a rough week. Sunday night into Monday, it snowed twenty inches of snow. The Tahoe which has the plow, was in the ditch most of the time, so Phillip and Jessie spent over seven hours getting it out just to have it slide back in again. It is heavy, wet snow and the Tahoe really needs new tires.

Finally, Tuesday morning the snow was crusty enough for me to drive the truck onto the center of the driveway. I got the driveway plowed and called the township to come and plow our road. I explained that I had to get Tom into town for his chemo treatments. They had the road plowed with the hour.

To our surprise, Tom's blood counts were high enough for him to receive his chemo. He will get his chemo on Tuesday. He is tired this week. Tom is still hanging in there even though he missed three days of work this week.

Thursday, March 17, 2006

Tom is worried that his employer is going to let him go. He is still covered under FMLA and he can apply for another twelve weeks next week. We are going to do this so he will not lose his job along with all our medical benefits. I can understand a company needing productive employees. Since Tom started work with the company, he has increased their profits greatly and improved their productivity. I think they at least owe him employment and benefits until he dies. We cannot afford COBRA and can use his short-term disability when he cannot work.

Friday, March 18, 2006

Tom fell on the deck again today. I could not get him up. I went inside and grabbed a chair. Between Tom and I we were able to get him up onto the chair and then into a standing position. I felt helpless as I watched him struggle for the least amount of energy to pull himself up. It is difficult to watch such a zealous man become so weak and helpless.

Saturday, March 19, 2006

Sandy and I spoke about their plans for moving. They want to come earlier then April, but financially they want to wait a few more weeks. I told Sandy that if it is too much of a heartache, that they should just wait. She assured me that it was important to her and Larry that they come to help. It would be nice to have her here. She is always so supportive having been my best friend since we were children.

Tuesday, March 21, 2006

Tom had the second session of cycle nine today. He is also receiving daily shots of GCSF and Erythropoietin to help increase both his white and red blood cells. His platelets have been low as well and are important to protect against excessive bleeding. His white and red counts are high enough today to continue with his chemotherapy. I will be learning how to give these shots to Tom, so we do not have to go to the hospital every day.

Wednesday, March 22, 2006

Tomorrow is Tom's birthday. I really thought that last year was going to be his last birthday. I am grateful that it was not. My gut tells me this year will be his last. We do need a miracle. I would like to live a longer life with Tom.

Thursday, March 23, 2006

Today is Tom's 52nd birthday. He made it another year. It has been rough for both of us. He is tired, having difficulty focusing close-up, difficulty reading and cannot seem to get enough sleep. His appetite is off again affecting his nutrition, which is affecting his blood counts.

I was so grateful for all the help Tom and I got when I was in treatment. Things are different with Tom in treatment. I had hoped Tom's side of the family could offer some help or support, but I guess their lives are too busy. They do not even come to visit Tom.

It is his birthday today and none of them has been to our house in over a year. We went to Gordon for Christmas otherwise we would not have seen them. I guess they are in denial that he will die soon.

I guess everyone figures I am healthy enough to handle it all myself, so the help from others is not there. I wish they could understand the truth about how I am doing in reality. I am in pain every day, very depressed and fed up with life.

Our son, Phillip, has been our main support and help. I am so grateful he is still living with us. I guess he delayed leaving home to help us through my cancer treatments and boom, we still needed him to help with Tom's.

The more Tom becomes dependent on me, the more tired I become. I must help him dress and undress. Get him whatever he needs when he needs it. He has so much trouble keeping his balance that I have to help him get up and down.

I am grateful to Phillip for all the daily help he is providing to both Tom and me. Rachel and Val come home on weekends to spend time with their dad, and I know this is important to Tom.

Lately, Tom is angry with me most of the time. I am not angry with him, as he no longer has control over it. I am angry at the situation. I am in such pain, and I know Tom does not notice it. He has his own problems. My legs still are not getting stronger as time goes by. Instead, they seem to be getting weaker. The hip pain is still almost unbearable when I put to much pressure on it. When I must use my body to help lift Tom, I can really feel how much I have not recovered.

I am discouraged about my own life. I am so tired and worn out. I hope this all passes. I hope one day I will feel like life is worth living. Right now, I do not.

Sunday, March 26, 2006

We decided to take Tom out for breakfast for his birthday celebration. We went to a restaurant in River Falls. This same restaurant sponsored several of the cars shows Tom and I had attended. I chose a Hawaiian theme since Tom always wore a Hawaiian shirt to work on casual Fridays. He is famous for his variety of Hawaiian shirts. Kathy, her husband, Gary, their two sons, Rachel, Valerie, their boyfriends, as well as Phillip and Jessie joined us. Our nephew Willie also helped us celebrate Tom's birthday.

The company was fantastic and the food wonderful. Tom was tired and tried to have a good time, but I think it was too much for him.

Cycle Four – Oral Chemotherapy
Monday, March 27, 2006

Today is day one of Tom's next cycle of Temozolomide oral chemotherapy. Tom is having a lot more difficulty walking. I told him to take the day off from work, but he wanted to go. I watched him walk into work, wondering if he was going to fall.

He managed to make it through the day, but I had to help him get into the car. I have noticed his co-ordination and balance are very poor these past few days.

Tuesday, March 28, 2006 – Oral Chemotherapy

As day two of oral chemotherapy began, I notice this morning that Tom could not walk very well at all. He managed to stand, but his legs would not hold him very well. There was no strength in his legs and no co-ordination. I suggested that he take a few days from work and get his strength back. I called into work for him. He had a doctor appointment, so I used that as his excuse.

We used the wheelchair to get Tom outside and then I helped him get into the truck. He is still able to pull himself up into the seat.

At his doctor appointment, we discussed his lower extremity weakness, which may be the result of developing Eaton Lambert Syndrome. This is an autoimmune disorder, which affects the calcium in the bones.

Cytopenia

Tom also continues development of cytopenia. Our bodies have three types of blood cells: white blood cells (WBC), red blood cells (RBC) and platelets. Cytopenia occurs when there is reduced production of any of those three types of cells. When the production of these cells is reduced, it can cause a other health issues. For Tom his blood cell count is very low, greatly affecting his platelets. Tom will continue to receive his daily shots of GCSF and Erythropoietin shots to hopefully increase his blood counts.

By this time, Tom has been on Temozolomide oral chemotherapy for four months.

I truly believe that yesterday was the last day that Tom will ever work again.

Eaton Lambert Syndrome
Wednesday, March 29, 2006 – Oral Chemotherapy

I learned how to give Tom his two blood building shots today. In past years, I have given vaccinations to hundreds of puppies. It is similar, but an eerie feeling to pierce human skin, especially Tom's skin. I did not want to be the cause of his pain. I am confident I can do this. The only hold up right now it that the insurance company has to approve me giving them to Tom at home. We have an authorization request in with them now.

Today was day three of oral chemo.

Thursday, March 30, 2006 - Oral Chemotherapy

This is day four of Tom's oral chemotherapy. Tom is having such a difficult time walking that he is using the wheelchair daily. I am relieved that both our bedroom door and the bathroom door accommodate the width of the wheelchair. It makes a big difference. This way Tom just has to slide from the chair either onto the toilet or onto the bed. It makes it much simpler for me.

Tom needs help to get in and out of a chair or the wheelchair and his weight is making my hips hurt all the time. Phillip or I wheel him into the bathroom, help him onto the toilet and then back up again into the wheelchair.

Phillip built a ramp on the front deck so I could wheel Tom to the Tahoe and help him get into the truck. I need to put my foot on the baseboard of the truck and put my knee under Tom's butt to help him up and into the seat.

I took Tom to the hospital today for an MRI of his brain. I got a wheelchair from the lobby to take him around the hospital for his tests. The tumors in his lung and in his brain have increased.

Oral Chemotherapy
Friday, March 31, 2006

It is getting more and more difficult to get Tom in and out of the truck. My sister, Val, said we could borrow her car to make it easier on Tom.

I have been giving Tom his two shots every day when we get to the hospital. We still do not have approval from the insurance company for me to give him these shots at home.

Tom is requiring more assistance with everyday needs. He continues to apologize for being so needy. I tell him he does not have to apologize for accepting help. I remind him of all the help he gave me when I was in treatment and that I am just returning the favor. This seems to ease his frustration. It was day five of oral chemo.

Saturday, April 1, 2006

Today I did a community garage sale at the Legion with Kathy and some other friends. Tom had purchased some electronic equipment last fall. The whole thing became a headache and a rip-off. The equipment was junk. The sellers have been arrested and waiting to go to trial. We had wanted to sell the items on-line, but it was all damaged or low quality. We decided to sell the items for pennies on the dollar to get rid of it.

My mom and dad came and spent the day with Tom. Lindalee and Jeff helped me at the garage sale.

Tom didn't miss me being gone so long that he called off and on all day. I felt badly that I was away from him for so long, but this was something that needed my attention.

The sale went well, and all the items were gone by the end of the day.

Sunday, April 2, 2006

Phillip's request for leave of absence from work is approved through FMLA. Starting Tuesday, he will be here all the time to help Tom and me.

Cycle Ten – Chemotherapy
Monday, April 3, 2006

At chemotherapy today, the nurse, Linda, had a rough time trying to get an IV started in Tom's arm. Tom asked if it were possible to get an IV port. Linda looked at me and I looked at her. She said to Tom, "I wish we had done that sooner."

We knew it was too late for that. It was too late because the surgery is to high risk, and he may not be around long enough to make the surgery worth the risk.

Tuesday, April 4, 2006

It was nice to have Phillip here to help me take care of Tom. Phillip made me an omelet for breakfast. Lately I have

183

been forgetting to eat breakfast, and often forget to eat through-out the day.

It is uncomfortable to watch Tom die. His eyes are bulgy, and he seems distance and separated from reality some of the time. He has not been able to walk for a week now. The MRI indicated that the tumors in his brain have multiplied and traveled to the frontal areas of his brain. This is causing Tom's inability to walk. Last week he would not eat or drink, became dehydrated, and entered the first stage of starvation. He had an IV to re-hydrate his system.

He gets very angry when I try to get him to eat or drink. I can emphasize with this. I remember when I was at that same point, so I realized how hard it is to make yourself eat when there was no desire or hunger present. He does not realize that he will die sooner if he does not at least drink water. His urine gets very dark orange as he becomes dehydrated.

Wednesday, April 5, 2006

Phillip and I tried to give Tom a bath today. It was awful. We managed to get him into the tub but could not get him out. We tried, tried, and just could not do it. Finally, after about twenty-five minutes, we were able to get him out. It was not only physically exhausting for all three of us, but it was degrading to Tom.

He tried so hard to get out of the tub and could not. It was another sense that he was losing his independence. This is the last time we will put him in the tub. I am going to get a shower bench to use. Between the two of us, I know we can manage to get him on the bench and out of the tub again.

If I had known better, this would have been the time to get home health care for Tom. I was confused about how it worked and I had not been given any advice on the subject.

If Phillip were not home each day to help me, I know I could not do it alone.

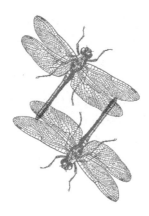

CHAPTER 13 - TOUGHER TIMES YET TO COME

Thursday, April 6, 2006

The toughest times are yet to come. Tom is deteriorating each day. The strength in his legs has not returned and he is in the wheelchair or a sitting chair all the time. He rarely tries to walk anymore.

I know that Tom is feeling tired, worn-out, and physically ill. He readily accepts help from me now. He no longer apologizes for needing the help he accepts.

It is getting tough. We have to lift him up or down for everything. He has bowel movements in his pants and last night in bed. It is extremely hard to clean up your husband like that. It reminded me of taking care of my babies. That is what Tom is becoming, a helpless child who has become completely dependent on me. It is a lot of responsibility.

When a loved one has a diagnosis of terminal cancer, the first thing you wonder is how long? That is a hard question to answer. It depends upon the individual person. The doctor mentioned nine to twelve months for Tom. It is fifteen months, and he is still fighting. His doctor is amazed at how long Tom has survived.

I know he is going to die soon, but he gave all he had to

live. There is no way to prepare for a loved one's death. I found this a good time to make sure I had taken care of the important things. Primary of course is proper medical and emotional support.

Then other area of importance is legal issues such as a living will, estate and personal wills. These are difficult things to think about, but Tom and I took care of this several months ago. I am relieved that we did, because at this time it would be even more difficult.

Medical Power of Attorney

Medical power of attorney is also important to have in place. It will contain all the details the patient wants, as they get closer to their death. A living will has limits and in some cases, a doctor can intervene on the patient's wishes. A Medical Power of Attorney gives all the patient's medical legal rights to the selected person or persons. This way the chosen person can carry out the dying person's wishes.

Memorial and Funeral Arrangements

Another area to consider is memorial and burial arrangements. I have been told it is less stressful to make most of the arrangements ahead of time when decision-making abilities are not hampered by grief.

It also gives the terminal patient the opportunity to specify their desires and wants for their final arrangements. I approached Tom by stating what I wanted for my final arrangements and simply asked him what his thoughts were for his. It seemed easier to discuss it as a conversation, so he didn't feel as though I had given up on his survival.

Get all of this out of the way as soon as possible. When all these things are in place, trying to make it through life after your loved one dies will be less stressful and less complicated.

It has been nine days since Tom has been to work. The way his health is going, I know for sure he will never return to work. Today at the doctor, this became more evident. His lower body weakness has increased, resulting from the progression of the metastasized tumors in his brain, as they continue to grow and multiply. The Cushingoid puffiness of his facial features is has become more prominent.

Tom will continue the Neumega, GCSF, and Procrit for his blood support. The Neumega is to support the growth of Palettes. Tom's voice has worsened, and the doctor believes it is thrush.

Friday, April 7, 2006

Tom's condition worsened suddenly. I realized his end is coming soon and I am shocked at how quickly it has arrived. I know it has been over a year, but it seemed to go so quickly. You do what you have to do each day. It is confusing, painful, and sad. The most important thing that I want to accomplish it to make the end of his days the best I can for him.

I need to remember to tell him that I love him as often as I can. I never let him feel guilty for needing help. We try to make it a team effort. I thank him each time he helps himself, so he has a sense of some independence left.

Saturday, April 8, 2006

We got a hospital bed with a tray table for Tom. It is too difficult to get him in and out of our bed and he spends most of his time in bed anyway. We put the bed in the living room. The kitchen, dining room and living room are all open to each other so Tom can be a part of everything that is going on at all times.

I moved part of the living-room furniture out but kept his big burgundy recliner. It is easy to move on the floor when he is sitting in it so we can turn him in the direction of either company or TV viewing.

I am sleeping on the floor in the living room next to Tom's bed. I am using a blow-up mattress so I can be nearby. Tom has a glass bell to ring when he needs something since his voice is no more than a whisper.

Monday, April 10, 2006 - Chemotherapy

While at chemotherapy today, Tom told the nurse, Linda, that he was going to ask Dr. H. if he could go back to work. Linda and I just looked at each other. We both knew that it was not going to happen but admired his determination.

Wednesday, April 12, 2006

I do not know how to express my feelings right now. There are so many feelings to sort. Taking care of Tom is sad and a lot of work. He is losing many of his abilities as the days go by. Having to hold his penis when he must pee and wipe his butt after he has a bowel movement is humbling and heart wrenching. I must change his wet clothes and soiled ones as well.

We need to wash him and change his bedding. I can see the sadness in Phillip's eyes as he helps me care for his dad. He quickly removes the bedding and goes straight to the laundry to wash them. He makes sure we have always at least two clean sets.

I promised Tom that I would take care of him to the end and that he could stay at home. Even though it is difficult to do, I will see it through to the end. I owe him that much. With Phillip's help, this is possible.

It is a lot of work taking care of a terminally ill person. His employer has not made it easy lately. Tom is still on FMLA (Family Medical Leave Act) which gave him twelve weeks of leave without a threat to his work.

The HR (Human Resources) at his work wants to terminate Tom's employment as soon as his FMLA is completed. I have discovered that Tom can take his three weeks vacation in the middle of his FMLA, which would extend it another three weeks.

If they do terminate Tom, we will lose all of his benefits. I think Americans With Disabilities Act may have some additional information I need to check out.

Tom has not received Social Security Disability and I am sure he will not live long enough for the determination of his eligibility. I applied for his disability in early March.

Thursday, April 13, 2006

Last night Tom soiled his bed. It was all over. It made my stomach upset. I hate this part most of all. I truly appreciate the change of bedding that Phillip keeps available at all times.

We have three sets of sheets to fit the hospital bed. When the girls were in the dorms, they had the extra-long sheets that are the same as a hospital bed. I never got rid of them, so they have come in handy.

I have been up since 4:30 this morning. I went to bed with a migraine and tried to ward it off. It is better, but with little sleep and more stress, I am surprised that I can function.

I am tired. I am tired of all the pain Tom is having. I am tired of him being so miserable. He does not seem to know he is as miserable as he is. He does not seem to know how dependent he is on others help. Yesterday he said he was going back to work because he did not want to lose his benefits. He does not realize that he cannot go back to work.

Tom's most recent MRI showed that the brain tumors have continued to grow and are spreading in the frontal area of his brain. This growth is causing lower body weakness and lack of control over bodily functions. Tom is now unable to walk. He can stand on his legs but cannot walk forward. His legs are getting weaker every day, but he is still full of hope.

His doctor changed his chemotherapy. Instead of both the oral and IV chemo, he is on just the IV chemo. Tom has exhausted all the chemotherapy drugs designed to fight lung cancer. Dr. H. is going to try a drug that has shown a small amount success with lung cancer. He will have IV treatments for four Mondays on and two Mondays off, then four Mondays on.

We go to the hospital every day for the injections because the insurance company would not authorize me to give them at home. It is getting harder and harder each day to get him there and Tom is getting weaker each day.

We have not given up. Each day he continues to survive is a chance for something new.

Friday, April 14, 2006

I am going to make an appointment with Tom's employer to discuss what their intentions are. I know if I talked to his boss, I would get the answers I need. I believe I can extend Tom's leave with ADA and apply for long-term disability right away. If not, to extend his short-term disability long enough to continue his benefits. If I understand the information correctly, it is Tom's option to substitute his three weeks' vacation in the middle of the FMLA to extend his employee status. I am not certain, and I will have to do more checking.

Phillip continues to make my daily omelet breakfast.

Saturday, April 15, 2006

Tom is using protective undergarment underwear continually because he has lost the sensation of having to go. He is in pain, cannot hear or see and his butt hurts. He does nothing but sleep. He will not eat or drink. It will not take long now if he gets no nourishment. He may survive a week. I fear it will not be longer than two weeks. I am going to call a priest on Monday. Tom has asked for his last confession and his last rights. That is important for Tom, as he is a faithful catholic.

I had a long talk with Lindalee, and she said it was time to let Tom go. Realizing that Tom is ready to go does not make it any easier.

Sunday, April 16, 2006

Rachel and Valerie came to visit Tom today.

Since Sandy and Larry were in the process of moving back here from Oregon, Lindalee, my niece Katie, and I were getting the small bedroom ready for them to use while they are here. We were also working on the garage so they could have a place to store their things.

Lindalee and Jeff have been coming over the last two Sundays. Jeff watched movies with Tom while Lindalee, and I cleaned.

I am going to talk with the oncology nurse and ask if we can stop the daily injections. Tom started going downhill with the platelet injections. I think the daily trips to town are too hard on him. If his blood improves, he can have the chemo, if not then he will not. I would like to talk Tom into stopping his chemo permanently and try to enjoy life as much as he can. I do not think there is any chance of remission or a cure, so it just seems like a waste of his health.

It has been hard to take care of Tom. He is heavy and lately, he is angry. He does not intend to be, but I am sure the pressure on his brain from the tumors is causing it. He is not drinking liquids and I told him I wanted to take him to the hospital to get an IV for dehydration.

He said, "I didn't know we were in trouble." I told him his urine was dark orange again, so he drank a can of Squirt and a glass of water. It is a start.

Decision to Stop Chemotherapy
Monday, April 17, 2006

Phillip came with us to chemotherapy because I could no longer get Tom in and out of the car on my own.

I decided to take the opportunity to go to the Funeral Home and talk to the director about arrangements for Tom. I wanted to have some information to share with Tom just in case he decided he wanted to talk about it.

I waited until Tom's IV was inserted and the chemo started before I left. Phillip stayed with him to keep him company.

I was gone about an hour.

By the time I got back, Tom got diarrhea so bad, and it would not stop. His nurse, Linda called Dr. H. and he said to discontinue the chemo treatment. It took over an hour to get the diarrhea under control. Linda continued IV fluids to help re-hydrate Tom due to the loss he was experiencing.

When we got home, the three of us discussed stopping his chemotherapy. Tom asked me if I thought it was a good idea.

I told him that it was beating up his body so much and was no longer affecting the tumors. I told him I felt he would have a better-quality life if he just did not have chemo for a while.

He agreed to stop for a while.

There were no more chemotherapy drugs designed to fight his type of cancer left, so it made sense to stop.

Tuesday, April 18, 2006

Tom, Jeff, and I went to meet with Tom's employer. I could tell from the expressions on his co-worker's faces, that they were shocked by Tom's condition. They seemed shocked by the appearance of his swollen and enlarged face and the wheelchair. The meeting did not result in a concrete solution, but with all we presented to them, we still had a guarantee of an additional four weeks of employment for Tom.

This at least gives me more time to figure out additional solutions to retain medical benefits without having to go on COBRA.

The girls are concerned about their father's survival. They tried to encourage me to do more research to find better ways to help Tom survive. I am so tired, and I do not have the energy to hunt down all the "cures" that might be out there. Tom has had the best treatment he can receive with the best doctor he could have, and I do not feel there is anything out there that will help.

It is not that I do not care, but I am tired. I have been at this for fifteen months, hoping and praying. I know the girls think I have given up on their dad.

I wrote them a letter.

It was as follows:

"I am tired and worn out. I get broken sleep and the physical stress on my body from lifting and helping your dad has worn me out."

"I have so many legal and medical battles to fight right now that mentally I am spread very thin. I am having a hard enough time just getting through each day that the thought of more research to help dad is very exhausting."

"I would like to think that there is hope for dad's longer life, but after watching him deplete over the past three weeks, I guess I have lost hope for his survival. I have not given up hope. I am just facing the reality that your dad is not going to survive."

"Don't be angry with me for these feelings as it may be the tiredness and stress that is talking. I love your dad very much and want to spend more time with him."

I have made so many adjustments with my life that it is

overwhelming. I am ignoring many of my needs to meet dad's first. I hope you guys understand. I know it is difficult to see the heart of another person, but please try."

Love, mom

Later that day they called and told me, they understood. This helped me immensely.

Wednesday, April 19, 2006

I spoke with Tom's brother Al, who has been in Alcohol Rehab since February and told him that Tom did not have much time left.

He was surprised since his brothers had been telling him that Tom was doing fine. I know it had been months since any of his brothers had seen Tom, so I had no idea how they could tell Al that Tom was doing fine.

"Believe me Al when I say he is going to die very soon. If you want to see him, you better come soon."

Al said he would see what he could do to get out. It was elective to stay in the rehabilitation, so I did not see any problem for him.

Later today, Marty and his wife came down from Gordon to visit Tom. Lynette worked with hospice care, and she was blunt with Tom and told him he was going to die soon. I knew the words were true, but I still did not want to hear them, and I did not want her telling them to Tom.

Lynnette and Marty expressed their concerns for Tom's spiritual life. Tom assured them that he was right with God. They prayed with Tom and then they left.

Thursday, April 20, 2006

Tom's urine was dark orange again. I called his nurse, Linda and she said to bring him in for an IV. On our way home, Tom said he never wanted to do that again. I asked him why and he just said, "Because I don't want it."

The he said he wanted to go to the casino. Phillip was not home because he wanted to spend some time with his girlfriend, Jessie, so I called Kathy.

I asked her if she wanted to help me take Tom to the casino. She said she would.

We only stayed for a short while because Tom was complaining that his testicles were burning. He was uncomfortable and I could see that he was not enjoying himself. We took him home.

Home Health Care
Friday, April 21, 2006

I called the local Home Health Care agency and arranged for Tom to have some home health care. I wish I had known more about home health services and what they could help with. I wish I had contacted home health care weeks earlier. We decided not to start Hospice care yet.

Home Health Care are health services provided to patients in their own home. Some of these services include medical and psychological assessment, wound care, medication teaching, pain management, disease education and management, physical therapy, speech therapy, and occupational therapy.

The primary goal is to provide reliable health care including medications and comfort for the patient while in the comfort of their own home.

Hospice care is very similar to Home Health Care with one major difference.

Hospice Care

Prior to hospice care, a patient can receive Palliative care. This is usually started between Home Health Care and Hospice Care. This care provides treatments for discomfort, stress, and relief from pain. Counseling may also be available with Palliative Care.

Hospice care is for terminally ill patients with less than six months to live. It also means the patient has accepted that they are going to die. Comfort care and immediate needs are met, but lifesaving treatments, such as chemotherapy is discontinued.

Hospice Care does not provide lifesaving treatments, such as CPR. Hospice care is treatment that concentrates on reducing the severity of the symptoms of the disease and let it continue its course. This is the reasoning behind discontinuation of treatments. The goal of Hospice care is to prevent and relieve suffering also to give dignity to the patient while dying.

Therefore, the main difference between Home Health Care and Hospice is that lifesaving treatments will continue during Home Health Care and are discontinued with Hospice Care.

The health care nurse came out to the house, and we discussed the services Tom could receive. She said an aid would come over tomorrow to help us bathe Tom. I thought that was a good idea.

After the nurse left Tom asked me," I'm not going to beat this, am I?"

I said, "I'm sorry, but probably not. I love you."

He said, "I love you more than anyone could ever love another person."

I know this is true.

We spend the next few hours talking.

He wanted to discuss the things he wanted done after he was gone.

He had me get a pen and paper. His voice was horse as he spoke, and I had to listen carefully. He had me list the three classic cars and the price I should sell them. He said I should sell the 429 Mustang to Phillip since he showed in interest in it. I told him I would.

He said if there was enough money, to pay as many medical bills I as could and any other bills that were left.

I was willing to do these for Tom, but I know he did not realize I had applied for Social Security Disability. I was not sure how my financial future was going to look like.

I kept all my medical problems from him. I did not want him to die thinking I was going to have ongoing medical concerns.

After discussing financial concerns, he asked me to write

some letters. The first three, though brief, were to our three children. Then he asked me to write one to my dad and to a few other people. It was difficult to write down his words because I knew his end was so near.

Suddenly he said he was hungry for a White Castle hamburger. I drove over to North St. Paul while Phillip stayed with Tom. I purchased every variety of White Castle hamburger they had and some onion chips and fries.

I was so excited when I got home as he ate one and half hamburgers and a handful of onion chips. It was good to see him enjoy some food.

At that time, I did not realize that the desire for favorite foods after being reluctant to eat, was a sign the end was near. Usually, three to four days before they die.

Al came over to the house shortly after that to stay for a few days. He had checked himself out of the treatment center. He told them that his brother was dying, and he wanted to spend time with him.

I got the impression that his brother, Dave, was upset with him. Dave had been instrumental to get Al into the rehab center and seemed upset that Al left early. If Dave were here, he would realize that Tom is close to death.

I am glad Al is here to help.

Saturday, April 22, 2006

Sandy called this morning to let us know they were leaving Portland and figured it would take about four days to get here since they were hauling the blazer with the rental truck on a trailer. I hope they get here on time to see Tom one last time.

When the woman from home health Care arrived to give Tom a bath, Al offered to help. I know Tom was reluctant to be bathed, but I was able to convince him that he would feel much better. He finally agreed.

Tom's condition continued to decline throughout the day. He would not eat. He lost all control over his urine and bowel movements. We were changing the bed more often throughout the day.

I could see that Phillip was experiencing a lot of stress, so I suggested that he take the night off and go out with Jessie for a while. He took me up on his offer. He did need to get away for a while.

I still cannot imagine what it is like to see your father in such a condition of helplessness and near death. I still have both of my parents and here is my son, helping his dad die with dignity.

He is a good son, and I am grateful that he is here to help us. Tom also looks forward to Rachel and Valerie's weekend visits.

I realize now that we should have begun Home Health Care when Tom was done with work. Home Health Care could have offered many services that may have made Tom's life much easier. I realize that some of these services, such as bathing would have made all of our lives much easier.

Sunday, April 23, 2006

Tom is much worse this morning. He was having difficulty breathing and was in an increased amount of pain. I contacted the Home Health Care nurse to come for a visit to assess Tom's condition.

After the nurse arrived and saw the level of Tom's pain and discomfort, she suggested that he change to Hospice Care. She also suggested he start the use of morphine to make him more comfortable. She tried to get a prescription for morphine filled for him, but with no success. She left and came back later with a bottle of liquid morphine and explained that the doctor will have a prescription of oral tablets filled on Monday.

She also had contacted an oxygen supply company because she felt that Tom needed help with his breathing.

Rachel and Valerie came over to visit with Tom today. He is having a difficult time talking. It is really a whisper. He blinks his eyes as response to a question. It takes a lot of energy for him to talk. His eyes are black and glazed and he seems to have difficulty focuses on things.

I overheard a brief conversation he was having with the

girls.

He asked them when they were graduating. They told him in three weeks. He was quite for a moment and then said, "I am sorry, but I don't think I will make it."

I know all of us wanted to cry to hear him say that. The girls just said, "Dad, don't worry. We are sure you will still be here for our graduation".

I did pray to God that if he could grant me any prayer that it would be for Tom to be able to see his daughters graduate from college. It is one prayer I really wanted answered.

Tom seemed to realize that his end was near. He did agree to the Hospice Care. He also told me that if his heart stopped, he did not want CPR. Tom said he was ready to go.

Home Hospice Care

This became the beginning of his hospice care. I remember wondering what hospice was all about but did not have any luck discovering the answer I needed. I wondered if I would know if the time was right and I wondered how the care would be provided. Once Tom went into home health care, the providers were instrumental in easing us into hospice care. It was then that I realized I did not need to worry about it once the process had begun, because experts in the field would be there to guide me along the way.

Essentially, when a person enters hospice care they have decided that any life saving efforts, such as chemotherapy in Tom's case, would end. It is the time when death is allowed to come and take Tom away but with grace and dignity.

Hospice care can be provided at home, a hospital, or a nursing home. Tom asked to die at home, so I was fulfilling his wishes.

Hospice care is the end-care of a person's life. Tom was now at the point when we knew that all hope for his survival was gone. Because this realization was now a reality, the most important thing now was to make Tom as comfortable and ease his pain as much as possible.

This brings up another issue that needed to be addressed when dying. His final wishes about not being resuscitated in the event he stopped breathing or if his heart stopped. Since he was ready to go, he decided that he did not want to be resuscitated. This is what is legally known as a DNR – Do Not Resuscitate.

After so many months of watching Tom receive treatments to save his life, it felt strange to watch him accept help designed to allow him to die. I could feel the fear of the end creep over me. I was not ready.

The oxygen service came late in the evening and set Tom up with the equipment. We were provided with detailed instructions on the use of the oxygen unit. This did help Tom, as he seemed more comfortable after the oxygen had begun.

Monday, April 24, 2006

Tom worsened through the night. Al and I took turns giving Tom his morphine every two hours.

The Home Health Care nurse came over early this morning. I explained to her that Tom wanted his last rights, but I could not find an available priest. She told me she knew a retired priest in New Richmond and would call to see if he were available. She left for a while. The news she shared upon her return was that a priest would be at our house within an hour.

It was very important to Tom to receive his last rights. I realized by now that Tom was ready to stop his fight against cancer. I think he realized that the cancer was going to win after all.

There was a knock on the door. As I opened the door, I sensed a strong familiarity of the priest standing there.

As I opened the door, the priest extended his hand and said, "Hello, I am Father Frayer."

I was so surprised!

"I can't believe it. I know you probably don't remember me, but you married Tom and me at St. Anthony's Church in Gordon, about 28 years ago."

He smiled and said, "I thought the name looked familiar."

Not only had Father Frayer married Tom and me, but he also baptized our three children. He was also the priest at the funeral of Tom's father. That was over twenty years ago.

Father entered our home and had a brief talk with Tom. They reminisced about Tom's parents and our marriage. Then he gave Tom his last rights. It was strange to sit as I watched my husband received his last rights. Last rights meant death. It was beginning to hit me that Tom was surely at the end of his days. Father Frayer officiated the beginning of our life together through marriage and now officiated the end of our marriage through death.

After Father Frayer left, Al got on the phone to his brother Marty.

He explained to him that Tom was not doing well and that he just had his last rights. Marty seemed to be in his denial stage but agreed to bring their mother down to our house to visit with Tom. From what I understood, no one had told Mary (Tom's mother), that the cancer had spread to his brain and that it was those tumors that were taking their toll on him.

Later that afternoon, Marty came with Tom's mom to visit. I could tell by Mary's expression, when she walked into the room, that she could not believe what she saw. She looked at the bed, the oxygen and Tom's state of health.

I could see her heart breaking in front of me.

Tom's communication was almost non-existent. He had little or no voice left and could not focus his eyes. Tom's cousin Joan, from Pennsylvania happened to call while they were still visiting. Even though the conversation with Tom was mostly one sided, Tom understood the love Joan was sending out to him.

Mary and Marty visited for a couple of hours and left for home. I wish they could have spent the night, but they declined.

Shortly after they left, my sister Sandy called. She said they were in Jamestown, North Dakota. I put the phone to Tom's ear while Sandy talked to him for a few minutes. Later Sandy told me she was assuring Tom that they would soon be there to help.

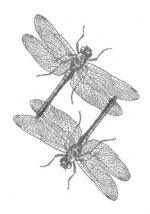

CAPTER 14 - UNTIL DEATH DO US PART

Tom's Journey Ends
Tuesday, April 25, 2006

I made an entry on the Caring Bridge web page at five o'clock this morning. I informed everyone that Tom has chosen to stop chemotherapy.

I also wrote:

"Tom has stopped eating and most recently, stopped drinking. He is on pain medication to help relieve the pain he began experiencing a few days ago.

It has been 15 months since he began his long battle with cancer, and I am afraid that his battle may be close to being over. I will update in a few days."

I sat near Tom for a while. He seemed to be having difficult time breathing, so I adjusted his oxygen.

I gave him his morphine at 7:00 a.m., and then waited to see how he was doing with it. I lay on the hospital bed next to him.

I kissed him and said, "I love you and I am going to miss you."

He blinked his eyes twice to let me know he understood.

I went into the bedroom to change my shirt. When I came

back into the living room, he had passed away. I was in total shock. Just a moment before he was still alive and moments later, he was not. I called down the stairs to Phillip and Al. They came immediately.

The two dogs, Rascal and Precious had been lying on the bed with Tom. When Al approached, they both stood up and snarled at him. It was heartwarming to know that they were protecting the body of their beloved master. I pet them both and set them on the floor.

Al checked Tom's breathing and confirmed he had died.

It was an eerie feeling to see his lifeless body lying on the bed. He looked like him, but the spirit that was his life had left his body. I hugged him, kissed him, and held him for a while.

Then I called our daughters and told them their father had died. They said they would be right over. I called my sister Lindalee and she said her, Jeff, and her son, Patrick (Tom's godchild) would be over as soon as they could get here.

Rachel and Val and their boyfriends, and Phillip and Jessie, were all together within an hour. Shortly, Linda lee and Jeff also arrived.

I called the funeral director and informed him that Tom had died. He asked me what time I wanted him to come to the house. We decided about eleven o'clock would be good.

Al called Tom's side of the family to tell them Tom had passed. Then I called the rest of mine.

Sandy and Larry were still on their way, in northern Minnesota. I felt so badly that they were not here soon enough to see Tom before he died. I called Sandy to let them know that Tom had passed away. Sandy cried and said she was sorry they had not made it in time.

I told her, "When you talked to Tom on the phone last night, he knew you were close. He just couldn't hold on any longer."

Once we were all together, we just sat near Tom and comforted each other.

I was standing behind everyone looking at Tom's lifeless

body, when I felt as though Tom was standing behind me and wrapped his arms around me in a big hug. I would like to believe this is true. It was comforting to know he had passed over and hugged me to take the love we had with him.

The fact that Tom had died had not hit me yet. I was doing the things I needed to do such as phone calls and talking with everyone.

I called Dr. H.'s nurse, Linda. I told her Tom would not make his appointment that morning because he had died. Linda expressed her sympathies and said she would tell Dr. H..

Within ten minutes, Dr. H. called. He expressed his sympathies as well. He told me he was impressed with Tom's strength and was surprised that Tom had survived as long as he did. Dr. H. continued to tell me that Tom was the most enduring and committed patient he had ever had. Dr. H. said he too, would miss Tom.

That really warmed my heart. Tom did fight a good fight and now he is peaceful and no longer in pain.

About eleven o'clock, the funeral director arrived at the house. He asked if we were ready for him to take Tom. I agreed.

Even though Tom was going to be cremated, the funeral director asked what clothes I wanted for Tom. It was amazing the great respect he showed for Tom's body. It was as though he were caring for a living person. It touched my heart.

I choose Tom's favorite salmon colored shirt that he had become quite attached to, his favorite jeans, his old leather shoes he loved to wear and a pair of black socks.

I place our wedding picture in the pocket of the shirt. Al gave a lock of his hair. He had long hair when he entered the rehab. When they cut his hair, he saved a lock of it for this purpose. Lindalee gave a rosary, and I added a motorcycle part. Our on-line selling of motorcycle parts was great fun for Tom, so I thought it appropriate.

The director wanted to know what I wanted done with his glasses. I told him that I wanted them donated. Tom and I had already decided that neither of us wanted our jewelry buried with us, so he did not wear our wedding ring. I put it away in my jewelry box.

Patrick helped the director lift Tom's body onto the gurney, ever so gently. Patrick is over six foot six inches tall and a very big person. It was touching to see how gently and lovingly he handled his godfather's body.

As the van doors closed and they drove away, I realized that Tom was gone forever.

Shortly after, everyone started taking all the medical equipment out of the house and into the garage. I called the suppliers and requested that they come and pick up their items as soon as possible. I wanted all of it out of my sight as soon as possible.

By three-thirty, Sandy and Larry arrived at the house. Their daughter, Angie, Tom's godchild had come with them. They also had a friend of Sandy's, Mary, who had come with to help with the driving.

Seeing Sandy gave my sadden heart a lift for a brief moment. Val and Rob joined us later that afternoon. Family members remained at the house until late into the night.

Wednesday, April 26, 2006

I slept in my bed last night. It was strange to think that Tom was not in the other room. I cried most of the night. I could not believe that Tom was gone. My entire body ached with sorrow.

We went to the funeral home today. I finalized the memorial and funeral arrangements. Tom specifically said that he did not want anyone to see him after he died. I am going to honor his wishes.

He wanted a Catholic funeral, and at our church, the presence of a body is required for ceremony. I selected a beautiful pine casket to embrace his body until his cremation after the funeral.

We selected the memorial cards and finalized the information that would go inside. The cover depicted trees that reminded me of the view out of our window when we look down upon the lake. It was perfect.

This was very hard to do, as it was yet another form of reinforcing that Tom had indeed died.

I am exhausted and worn out. I am not ready for the memorial or funeral. Sandy and Larry are moving their possessions into the garage. They have to return the moving van tomorrow, so it needs to be unloaded. Their bedroom needs to be set up. I would like to have Tom's memorial next week and the funeral the following day.

I selected Tuesday, May 2 for the memorial at the local Funeral Home and Wednesday, May 3 for the funeral at our local Catholic church. Father Frayer volunteered to do a prayer session at the memorial Tuesday evening. That warmed my heart.

Thursday, April 27, 2006

I wrote the following entry in the caring bridge web page.

"It is with great sadness that I share with all of our friends and relatives.

Tom passed away in our home on Tuesday. I am in awe of his strength and tenacity that Tom showed during his long fight against cancer.

He started experiencing body pain last week but was comfortable before that. He had not eaten for a few days, but on Friday, he asked me to get him some White Castles. I drove to N. St. Paul and came home with every variety plus onion chips, fries and mozzarella sticks. He ate two burgers, the jalapeño one first. It was good to see him enjoy one of his favorite foods.

He visited with family on Saturday and Sunday, the one thing he really wanted, his family around him. Monday, he became less aware. He started on pain medication on Sunday, which gave him comfort the two days that he remained with us.

Moments before he passed, I kissed him, told him I loved him. He moved his eyes slightly, which was his way he let us know he understood. Moments later, Tom passed from this world to the next.

Tom is greatly loved and will be greatly missed by all of us.

I wish to thank everyone for all the love and support that you have shown Tom and our family throughout the past 20 months."

It was the last entry I made on the web site.

I finalized the Obituary wording today and decided which newspapers the obituary would appear. These will include papers in Northern Wisconsin since that is where Tom spent most of his youth. I also choose Menomonie because Tom spent a few years of his life there while attending college and graduated from UW Stout.

It is amazing how networking can be so effective. Tom had worked at three companies in this area over the years. Almost immediately, the engineers of the varied companies had all begun to email each other to share the sad news of Tom's death. I knew Tom had been well liked, but this confirmed my thoughts.

Friday, April 28, 2006

All of the condolences' we received from so many people was heartwarming. Friends dropped by with prepared food and food supplies. There were so many people stopping by that it became a whirlwind for me. It was also a whirlwind for Sandy and Larry after having done so much traveling.

I could feel all the energy leave my body as I tried to cope with the loss of Tom. Even though I knew it was inevitable, I am in total shock that he is gone. It is surreal. The love of my life is gone.

The medical equipment is still in the garage, and I wish they would all come and get it. It is a painful reminder that I do not need. Phillip took down the ramp today. I am relieved to see it gone as well.

Saturday, April 29, 2006

My cousin, Bob, came for a visit. He stayed most to the day, reminisces about the past. I remember telling him at my grandmother's funeral that we needed to get together when it was not a funeral. However, here we were visiting because of another death.

It was good to see him.

Sunday, April 30, 2006

Someone left a small booklet at the house and while I was reading it, I wished I had read it much sooner. The booklet is "Gone From My Sight" by Barbara Karnes. It simply explains the process of dying and if I had read it sooner, I would have noticed certain indicators that Tom's time was nearer than I had thought. When you decide to put a loved one into Hospice Care, be sure to get a copy of this booklet. I highly recommend it.

Monday, May 1, 2006

I had started to pack Tom's clothes into boxes a few weeks ago. I was not in the frame of mind to do anything with them today, so I put them into the back of the closet. I decided that I did not want to sort through his things after he died. I knew it was the right choice for me. I can deal with them later.

Memorial Visitation
Tuesday, May 2, 2006

I chose the blue dress with dark blue flowers to wear to the memorial. It was one of Tom's favorite dresses, so I decided to wear it. My hair was still quite short, so I did not have to fuss with it.

My dad called and said that mom was not feeling very well. Mom has been sick for a long time. I wish the doctors could find out what is wrong with her. Dad said they would try to make it to the memorial.

We went to the memorial without them.

Some co-workers of Tom's offered to serve a small luncheon for the guests at the memorial. I was very grateful to them.

I had completed the memorial picture boards the week before Tom died. Lindalee had come over and helped to finish them. I placed our wedding album out on a table for people to view.

On top of the very serene pine casket, I placed several pictures of Tom housed in matching pine picture frames. I nestled the stuffed pink panther toy I had given to Tom before we were married among the pictures.   The pink panther became our favorite character when Tom and I were dating, and I kept the toy all these years as a memento.

The flowers were beautiful and framed the setting with peace and tranquility.

Sandy, Larry, and their children, Eric, and Angie sent a baby apple tree instead of flowers. It is so cute. This was to honor Tom and his love for trees. He planted two apple trees on our property when we first moved in. Each year thereafter, he would make apples pies from our own apples. It touched my heart at their thoughtfulness.

Tom's mother and brothers came before the memorial began. It was good to see them. After a while, I began to lose track of all the people who had come. I found a place to sit and let people come to me. I was so tired and wanted to rest. Some people I remember seeing and others I do not.

Sandy informed me that over 250 people had stopped to offer their last respects to Tom. Yes, he was loved.

Mom and dad arrived at the house after the memorial was over. Family members also gathered at the house, and everyone ate pizza. Mom was still not feeling well, so she slept. I hope mom is better tomorrow, as dad is one of the pallbearers. That was one of Tom's wishes. After Tom's father died, Tom adopted my dad as his own. They had a great relationship.

Tom's Funeral
Wednesday, May 3, 2006

Mom was still too ill to go to the funeral, so my niece, Julia and husband, Dave volunteered to stay with her during the funeral. Even though mom was so sick, it was important for my dad to go to the funeral. He had to say his goodbyes to Tom.

Tom and many of his flowers were already at the church when I arrived. Everything looked lovely and peaceful. I was pleased. Phillip, Rachel, and Valerie sat in the front pew. I sat next to them and then Tom's mother, Mary, sat next to me. Since she was Tom's mom, I felt we should sit together.

We sang the songs I had chosen, and the priest read the scriptures I had chosen. When it came time for the Eulogy, our three children and I went to the podium. I had written a eulogy for Tom, and I wanted to read it. I asked Rachel if she would finish it, I could not get through it. She agreed.

Tom's Eulogy

"It is amazing how a single word can change your life. Words like birth, marriage, divorce. For our family, one of the most powerful words that changed our lives was cancer.

As many of you know, our lives for the past twenty months, has been centered around cancer. Only five months after my diagnoses, Tom got his. We both had the same radiologists and oncologist and many times our appointments were for both of us. It would seem almost romantic if it were not so serious."

"However, dealing with caner showed us how strong our marriage was. You may think that these past twenty months have been nothing but worry, concern and sadness, but surprisingly enough, those months were full of love.

Full of Tom's great love for me, as he nurtured and supported me, through my cancer care. He was loving, kind and understanding. He held my hand through my tears, vomiting and pain. He took very good care of me. Being a caregiver is an act of love.

Tom was strong for me when I was weak. His support, faith and strength were the key to my survival.

Tom continued with his great love for us through the tenacity and endurance he showed as he fought his own cancer. My cancer experiences proved to be a form of confidence during Tom's treatments. He would ask me, "Am I supposed to feel this way?" "Is the chemo causing this?"

"His long journey through cancer was also a time for him to express his love for his family, as he realized that he was going to die. Fighting his cancer, as long and as hard as he did, was

Tom's greatest act of love. He wanted to survive so he could continue to take such great care of his family, of which he had done
all of his life."

"When he was still able to, a day never went by that he
did not tell me he loved me. One of the last things he said was
that his family being around him was the most important thing
to him. His family has always been the most important thing
to him. He had hopes of someday being independently wealthy,
as most of us do. However, even without the monetary wealth,
Tom told me he was the richest man in the world because of his
family."

"During all of the treatments and doctors and such, we
found many times to make memories. He was relieved that I
had survived my cancer. We made it to Oregon to visit Sandy
and Larry, where Tom was able to experience a dream he had,
of ocean fishing. We were able to enjoy a mini vacation to Las
Vegas. He knew his daughters were about to graduate from college, something very important to him."

"The five years before cancer entered our lives, no two
people could have asked for a better life together. Tom was
pleased with his job, something that was second only to his
family. We spent many hours together over a two-year period
restoring a 71 Mustang. Even though the car won many award
trophies, the time we spent together was the greatest award of
all. Over the past 12 years, we never missed watching a Packer
game together."

"Tom had a dynamic personality. He was very dedicated,
whether it was family, his work, Boy Scouts or hobbies. He gave
100% and often more to whatever he did. He never gave up,
even when things seemed dim, not in his love, family, work, or
his fight against cancer. The cancer has taken Tom away from us
in his physical form, but the cancer cannot take away his spirit.
Tom is now free of the limitations the human body has on the
spirit. He is free of pain and suffering. He is waiting for me and
when my time comes, we will find each other."

"I am very blessed to have had Tom for a husband and

such a wonderful father to our children. A few days before he passed, I asked him if he would wait for me in heaven. He smiled and said, "Who else would I wait for?" That was love. That was Tom."

After the funeral, the pallbearers lovingly placed the casket containing Tom into the van where it returned to the funeral home to await his cremation.

The women of the church set out a wonderful lunch and we went downstairs to gather for good conversation. To my surprise, my best friend Rachel (my daughter Rachel's namesake) was there. I cried when I saw her, both with joy and sadness.

It was a time for tears as Tom's brothers realized that their brother was gone. I knew their pain as it was my pain also.

Later, friends and family gathered at the house to tell happy stories about how Tom and celebrated that he had lived.

Thursday, May 4, 2006

Rachel and Valerie had their senior art shows at UW Stout in Menomonie today. My sisters all came to the show to help honor their accomplishments. As I looked at the beautiful paintings and graphics, Rachel had designed, and the amazing metal sculptures and jewelry Val had created, I missed Tom. I wished he could have been there to see how talented his daughters are.

I feel he was there in spirit and know he was aware of his daughters' gifts.

Friday, May 5, 2006

I am still in shock that Tom is gone. The last of the medical equipment left today. I was irritated that it took so long for it to be picked up. I still expect Tom to ring his bell and want something from me, but I know he is not here, and I miss him so very much.

Fund Raiser
Saturday, May 6, 2006

Rachel, Valerie, Kathy, and Sandy continued with the fundraiser that had been set up before Tom died. I wanted to cancel it because I was not up to it, but everyone said it was for the best because of the enormous medical bills I could not pay. I reluctantly agreed.

I am glad I agreed because people who could not attend either the memorial or the funeral came and offered their condolences.

The DJ Kathy got for the fundraiser was one of my and Tom's former Boy Scouts, David. It was nice to see him after so many years.

He was looking at the memorial picture boards and pointed to a picture of Tom shortly before he died.

"Who is that? He asked.

"Tom, just before he died", I replied.

"Oh, my gosh," he said, "he looks so different".

I explained to him all the medications he had been taking and they greatly affected his appearance.

Dave was a great DJ and kept things going for the day. Lindalee, Jeff, and Al came to help as did our three children. It was an emotional day for me. I do not know how I got through it. All around me were reminders that Tom was gone. It was very difficult.

Sunday May 7, 2006

We planted Tom's memorial apple tree today. It is sitting under the spreading arms of an original apple tree that Tom had planted. Tom would have been very pleased.

Monday, May 8, 2006

The funeral director called to tell me that I could pick up Tom's ashes. Once I brought them home, I needed to decide what to put the ashes in for the internment in Gordon. Larry had a vintage wine box from an Oregon winery. I thought that would be appropriate since Tom enjoyed our tours of the vineyards while we were there.

To this box, everyone added a special item that signified the things Tom enjoyed in life. I purchased a small personal sized silver urn with a nice blue design on it, for some of Tom's ashes so I could keep them with me. Blue was Tom's favorite color.

I decided to pick May 19 for the internment. It was our wedding anniversary, and I could not think of a better way to make it through that day, then to have Tom's internment. It would be like doing something special with him. It seemed like a special way to say goodbye.

Social Security Denial
Tuesday, May 9, 2006

I got a denial for Social Security Disability for me today. I am going to file an appeal. Filing for disability is difficult for me. I must admit that physically and mentally I am not the same person. I have to adjust to physical limitations that I am finding difficult to accept. I have always been very physical, and it is an emotional struggle to learn to accept these limitations.

I still experience great physical pain when I walk, and it seems to be getting worse instead of better. I still do not have the bladder control I want. I am adjusting little by little to wearing protective undergarments. I am still constantly concerned about having a bowel attack, especially in public.

Wednesday, May 10, 2006

Today I celebrated my 52nd birthday without Tom. It was the first birthday in over twenty-nine years that I spent without him. I was sick and lay on the couch most of the day. I developed a pain in my side a few days ago, and still have it. Everyone wants me to go to the doctor, but I do not think I could walk into the hospital right now without totally breaking down. There are too many memories for me there.

Thursday, May 11, 2006

Today Val had her "Artist in Residency" showing at UW Stout in Menomonie. This honor is very exciting, and she has been working on her display for the past several months.

Sandy and I went to her showing together. Lindalee and Jeff went also. I was very proud of her. She also received a publication in which her profile and artwork were featured. She gave a copy to me to take home.

Once we got home, I reached into the back seat for Valerie's publication. As I reached for it, I thought, "I can't wait to show this to Tom". Then I remembered that I could not.

Friday, May 12, 2006

I am still not feeling well today with a lot of pain in my right side. I have not been to the doctor because I am waiting until after the girls' graduation. I am having difficulties walking so Sandy said she would push me in the wheelchair at the girls' graduation tomorrow.

Rachel and Valerie's College Graduation
Saturday, May 13, 2006

I pulled myself together and put on a happy face to celebrate the girls' graduation. Marty brought his mother, Mary. My parents and immediate family attended also. I was pleased that they came.

I spent most of the graduation ceremony crying. My thoughts were of Tom. It seemed so awful to me that he missed this great event by only three weeks. I was so proud of our daughters. After their graduation ceremony I hugged them both and said, "I am so grateful that you did not defer your last semester. Your dad knows that you both did graduate. It is the best gift they could have given him."

We all went out to eat and had an enjoyable afternoon. When I think of it though, I feel badly that their celebration could not have been more festive. Tom and I planned a big party and we had considered giving each of them a car for graduation. It is amazing how plans can change so dramatically.

Even though the celebration did not happen as planned, I know that Tom is proud of his two daughters as they walked across the same stage that he had twenty-eight years earlier.

Hospitalization - Rita
Tuesday, May 16, 2006

Sandy and Larry took me to the emergency room late last night. The pain in my side has gotten worse. After spending a few hours in ER, the doctor decided to admit me. I had an enlarged appendix, and I was severely dehydrated. My blood showed signs of malnutrition as well.

My personal doctor, of whom I had not yet replaced because I had been seeing Dr. H., decided to run more useless tests. I was still angry with her since she did nothing about the lesion that developed into cancer. I no longer had faith in her. She was looking for more cancer. Dr. H. came by and assured me that there was no cancer. I guess he could not understand why my personal doctor was even looking. My guess because she missed my cancer the first time, she wanted to protect herself.

My blood counts were low which I think may have been because I had not been eating very well the past few weeks. I believe my condition is a result of my grieving. Grieving directly affects the health of your body. It interferes with you sleep, eating and heightens your stress level. I know I was not drinking enough water and food did not interest me. That is saying a lot. Even though I only weight about one-hundred and forty pounds at five-foot nine, I love to eat.

Wednesday, May 17, 2006

My side is feeling better and all I want to do is get out of the hospital. I don't understand why my doctor won't let me get out.

Thursday, May 18, 2006

I tried to let my personal doctor know that I needed to get out of the hospital today because Tom's internment is tomorrow. It seems she never got my message. Late this evening when she was making her rounds, I told her I wanted to go home. She said she wanted to keep me another day.

Finally, when I explained to her how important tomorrow was, she reluctantly let me go home.

Tom's Internment
Friday May 19, 2006

Early this morning I had to go to the clinic. I had another bladder infection. It is sad that my doctor kept me in the hospital for three days and could not even find a bladder infection. I started antibiotic the bladder infection again.

Today would have been my and Tom's twenty-seventh wedding anniversary. Today we will place Tom's ashes into the earth.

I miss Tom very much. There is a void in my life. I expect him to come through the door any time. I find myself saying, "I can't wait to share this moment with Tom." I missed him at the girl's graduation.

I am full of should a, would a, and could a. He died sooner that I had imagined. I thought maybe June, but that did not happen.

I gathered the things I wanted for the internment in Gordon. Plastic wine glasses and a couple bottles of Lambrusco wine. We served this wine at our weeding twenty-seven years ago today.

I rode with Sandy and Larry. Our children all rode together. Halfway up to Gordon, I realized I had forgotten to get flowers for Tom's grave. We stopped in Cumberland at the floral shop we have used many times in the past.

My sister explained to the woman that I needed flowers for my husband's internment and that today would have been our 27th anniversary. I thought she was going to cry. She created one the most beautiful bouquets I have ever seen.

We made it as far as Spooner when I decided that I also wanted flowers for Tom's dad's grave and for my Uncle John's. Once again, the entire story of our events and the anniversary internment was told, and once again, everyone at the shop was teary eyed. They made beautiful small arrangements, one for each grave.

Mary, Marty and his wife, my parents, Lindalee, Jeff and Patrick and our children all arrived at the cemetery. A hole, the correct size for the box, was waiting, covered with a green grass mat. I gently placed the wine box containing Tom's ashes into the ground. Using the small shovel, which had been left for us, I place the first bit of dirt upon the box. My children followed me and then anyone else who wanted.

We stood around drinking the wine or juice for those present that did not drink, thinking about Tom. He was two plots from his dad. At least he is near his dad, something he wanted. The two plots next to his parents were Al's, but he gave up the second for Tom and I. I tried to do all the things we had talked about before he died. He also requested that on his gravestone all he wanted was "Tom", not Thomas John.

It was difficult to see the small mound of dirt and realize that Tom was truly gone. It was such a difficult concept to grasp. It seemed so sad to leave Tom there. There was not even a headstone yet.

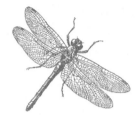

CHAPTER 15 - BECOMING A WIDOW

There is no experience in life that can prepare you to become a widow. It is a transformation from having been a couple to becoming a single. It is a sense of loss that you cannot even imagine. One day you are sharing your life and dreams with your spouse and the next you are trying to understand why you are now alone.

After Tom died, well-wishers told me that the pain I feel from his loss would lessen with time. The way I feel right now, I find that hard to believe. The first six months after Tom died were many hours and days full of tears, confusion, grief, guilt, and loss.

Letters to Tom

I missed my daily conversations with Tom. He was my sounding board and talking with him served to help me sort out decisions and choices I had to make. My journal entries become daily letters to Tom. This gave me a sense that I was still connected to him. The writing become daily conversations with him, even though they were one sided.

As I wrote my entries, I was not pretending that he was still alive, just hoping that somehow my thoughts and ideas would still reach him in his afterlife. The entries served to ground my life in a way that seemed tangible and comforting.
Tuesday, May 23, 2006

"Dear Tom, It has been four weeks since you left. I have

missed you every day. It is hard to believe you are gone. I miss your smile, I miss the way you said my name, I miss everything about you.

I hope your passing was a peaceful one. Phillip and I did all we could to make things good for you. You went so fast. I was not ready. I am sorry I was not beside you when you died. It was only a few minutes, that was all, only a few minutes.

I wish I had sat by you more often. I am grateful we had talked on the Thursday and Friday before he died. It gave me peace to know we talked about so many things I had wanted to talk about the months before you died. Thank you for the good life you gave me, the home, love, and friendship.

I am sorry for all the times I may have hurt your feelings. I hope I gave you a good life. I know you loved me more than any mortal could love another with your whole heart and soul.

Thank you for being my love." Rita

Even though we had the opportunity to talk before Tom died, it did not make accepting his death any easier. The moment he died was still a shock. One moment he was here and the next moment he was gone.

I believe that knowing someone you love is going to die and you have time before it happens does not make it any easier. A profound emptiness replaces your loved one's presence the moment they are gone.

PET/CT scan - Positron Emission Tomography
Thursday, June 1, 2006

The weeks that followed Tom's death was full of difficult adjustments. I still had to deal with my health issues. My personal doctor wanted me to have a PET/CT test. I am not certain why, maybe to make sure the cancer treatments were successful.

A PET is a Positron Emission Tomography, which utilizes nuclear technology to create images of the internal body. The PET scanner tube remaindered me of a large donut, like the tube shape of a CT scanner.

Radioactive tracers are injected into your body. I was a little intimidated when the technician came into the room in a hazardous chemical suite. He had a canister of which he opened and removed a syringe with the radioactive tracer. The tracer is more rapidly absorbed by malignant tissues than by normal tissues. The scan detects the areas of the body where the tracer has a higher level of absorption indicated possible disease.

After the injection, I had to lay still for about 30 minutes so the tracers can be absorbed by your body. I was concerned about having to go to the bathroom since I had poor bladder control. The technician said that I should lie still for as long I could. I managed to make it for the 30 minutes.

After going to the bathroom, I lay on a moving table and was slide into the donut shape scanner. I have claustrophobia, so I found this uncomfortable. As the scanner began, I could feel a heat throughout my body. There was no discomfort from the test but laying still for such a long amount of time was. I had my hands above my head, which caused pain in my neck from my previous spinal deterioration.

The claustrophobia took over and I wanted out. I cried until the exam was complete.

My PET was done in conjunction with a CT (CAT scan). The two tests act cooperatively, providing more detailed information than can be obtained if the two tests were done separately. PET can also be done in conjunction with an MRI.

Monday, June 18, 2006

Jessie moved in with Phillip. I like having Phillip still live here so I am happy that Jessie feels comfortable about moving in with us. Even though the house is full of family, I find that I hide in my bedroom most of the time. I think of Tom every day and when I think of him, I find myself crying. It seems like I cry ten times a day.

Tuesday, June 20, 2006

I am looking forward to the day when I no longer had to have semi-annual exams. The PET scan indicated that the tumor has not redeveloped. Like many cancer patients, I live in fear that my cancer will return. I had gone through so much to defeat it, but I still felt vulnerable to its former hold on me.

However, the cancer is not the main focus of mine. My main focus is trying to understand how I am going to continue living without Tom.

A grief support group would be beneficial for me at this time or self-help books on dealing with grief would be a good idea. I know this, but I do not want to turn to any of these resources right now. I feel exhausted and the idea of having to find a support group sounds like a lot of work.

Living Other People's Lives

Instead of facing my own life, I realize I am keeping my mind distracted by being involved in other people's lives, so I could avoid thinking about my own.

My sister Sandy and I finally talked my parents into selling our childhood home, which has been rental property since 1976. It needs painting, cleaning and repair. I am not sure if I am physically up to this challenge. I am still paranoid about bladder and bowel accidents. I feel embarrassed when it happens, even though I wear undergarments most of the time, accidents still happen. At least it will be just family helping with the house.

I am being cautious while working on the house, but I find that my legs and hips still hurt, and I experience fatigue. While I do drink plenty of water to avoid dehydration, my appetite has not yet returned. My sisters and father make sure I eat. Treatments and depression may be contributing factors to some of these conditions.

The work does serve as a distraction from my real life. With such a varied number of thoughts tumbling around in my head, distractions allow me to avoid putting them into perspective. The biggest thought was my guilt that I survived, and Tom did not.

My life is upside down. I feel out of place in my life and my home. Even with others around me, I feel lonely without Tom. The presence of others living in my home requires me to adjust to lifestyles and routines that are so different from the ones Tom, and I had. The biggest adjustment is Tom's absence.

When I take a moment to stop and think about my life, the loneliness and sense of loss is overpowering. I cannot see my life without Tom. I wanted Tom and my old life back.

Tuesday, June 27, 2006

"Dear Tom, I am so enjoying this morning. Sandy and Larry are gone for a few days. It is peaceful and quiet. I had coffee alone, watched what I wanted on TV and really enjoyed the morning. I wish you were here with me. I don't know how to move on with my life.

Life is strange when your spouse dies. It is not easy at all. I have no one to talk with, you know, from my heart. If I try to talk to others, they are unintentionally critical or mean, or full of impractical advice, or they just do not understand what I am trying to express.

I am lonely without you and feel as though I have no special friend. I miss you and love you. Rita"

Saturday July 1, 2006

Mom asked if I would help with the annual Fourth of July brat sale in Gordon. My first thought was to say no, but she counted on my help each year. It was for a good cause, so I agreed. When the muscle cars roared by during the parade, the sounds of the high output engines made me sad. Tom was not among the drivers in the parade and my heart knew it. It will be a long time, if ever, before I will be able to take pleasure in a fine classic muscle car.

Wednesday July 6, 2006

Work on the house in the cities continues. Often, I feel frustration because I cannot work at the same pace and endurance as in the past. I tire easily and take frequent breaks. It is nice to know the "boss" so well, since my seventy-four-year-old dad has to rest almost as much as I do.

Spiritual Beliefs

I harbored a strong anger against God. I feel that it was unfair that God took Tom away from me. I survived cancer so we could spend our lives together. Tom's life was a vital part of my life. Tom had such a great future of which he had worked his whole life to obtain now it is gone. I do not know how I feel about God anymore. I do not believe in Him the same way I did before Tom's death. Tom's death changed my perspective on the Devine, life, and death.

When a loved one dies, some people's faith in God is strong enough to carry them through their times of grief while maintaining their belief in God and his plans for them. I on the other hand, responded like many others, and I am filled with questions about my beliefs.

I can take comfort in knowing that Tom passed on with his faith in God as strong as it had been throughout his life. My difficulties may not be due to lack of faith, but pure anger, anger at God. Of course, I cannot blame God for all the evil in the world, but I can be angry with Him for a while.

Tuesday, August 1, 2006

"Dear Tom, my life is lonely without you. I am confused and lost. I do not trust anyone and feel guarded about opening my heart. I missed you so much. I still cry every day, feeling so alone, and so lost. I wish you were here; I wished you could come back and talk to me just one more time. Love and miss you, Rita."

I still cannot figure out what I will do with my life. My state of limbo is as strong as it was the months before Tom died only now, I am alone. As I remember the times when I had wished it were over, I really regret having said those words. I was not in a hurry for Tom to die; I was in a hurry for him to get better, for him to survive.

I knew from the beginning that he would not. I was thinking about how things could have been different. If I had not been in cancer treatment, we may have found out about Tom's cancer sooner and maybe he could have survived or at least survived longer. If his doctor had looked further when he came in with the persistent cough in September, could he have found the cancer soon enough to have prolonged Tom's life?

I am grateful to Tom for his determination and drive, giving us fifteen months longer together. I did not realize all the pain he was in until months later when I looked at the last pictures of him. Even through the camera lens, it was evident that he was struggling each day. I guess I was so caught up in his care and my recovery, that I did not see his intense pain. I did not notice how dramatically his looks had changed from all the medications. I felt a tinge of guilt that I had wanted him to live a little longer. I did not see that he was ready to go.

Wednesday, August 9, 2006

"Dear Tom, there is a cricket in the house. It is supposed to be a good omen, to bring good luck. I am one-step closer to my disability. Sandy and Lindalee are helping with the paperwork. Since I had treatments, it is confusing for me to organize my thoughts in a presentable way.

I am working on getting a headstone. I am sorry I did not get to it sooner. I promise to have it placed by the end of the month. I miss you!"

My life's distraction continues with work on the house in St. Paul. Work is slow but sure, one room at a time, one problem at a time. As the days pass, the house looks cleaner and repaired. My body is holding up for now, but I am feeling more and more tired each time I help. Adjusting to my new physical limitations and endurance are still difficult for me to accept. My hips hurt more each day and the fatigue catches up to me frequently. My mind and spirit want to do the physical things that my body can no longer handle and become emotional conflicts that I need to work out.

Alcohol Detoxification – Tom's Brother Al

Time continued to progress along its way and the days turned into months after Tom's death. I continued to avoid my own life by being involved with other people's lives.

Sunday, September 17, 2006

"It's been about five months, Tom, but it hasn't gotten any easier. The loneliness is getting stronger each day. Al is still struggling with his alcohol addiction.

I took him to alcohol detoxification at the hospital today. He was having a rough time. I am afraid that his alcohol problem will always be a part of his life. I am trying to keep my promise to you, help your brother, but I am not as strong as everyone thinks I am. I struggle every day to make it through.

While I was in the room with Al at the hospital, I looked at him, and he reminded me of how you looked just before you died. Death was all over Al's face.

I looked at Al and said, "I will never do this again. Right now, you remind of Tom before he died and I cannot handle this anymore."

He did not reply, but I know in my heart that I cannot be Al's support for this anymore.

I know Al relied on you quite a bit and I have tried to take your place, but I cannot. I will continue to do my best with Al, but I can only do so much. He will always be my brother.

I am still very sad and lonely and miss you as much as you loved me. Love, Rita"

Monday, September 25, 2006

Even after five months since Tom passed away, I still ached so much when I remember that day. There is emptiness in my chest. It is my heart aching. I feel a loneliness I have never felt before and it is the first time I really feel alone. It is very hard, to be alone. Tom was my friend, my husband and lover. He was a major part of my life. Everything is different.

The routines, the surprises, and the adventures we shared are all gone. My life changed as much as Tom's; except I did not die.

I think by keeping busy with dad's house has helped me to make it through these past months, but I know that soon the house will be complete and sold. The time has come for me to think about my future and not rely on other people's needs to help me get through each day.

My challenge now is to start living my life again. I know Tom would want me to be happy. I started taking a new anti-depressant and I continue to work on quitting smoking.

Thursday, September 28, 2006

The house in the cities sold and it is a day for celebration. We are very proud of our accomplishment. I realized it was time for me to work on my life by developing goals and plans for my future. I signed up for a grief support group scheduled to beginning the end of October.

Mom's Heart Attack
Friday, October 13, 2006

Circumstanced have put my life on hold once again due to other people's needs.

Dad called Sandy and I because he was worried about my mother's health. He wanted us to come to Gordon and to help him with her. When we arrived, she was lethargic and weak. Somehow, we managed to get her into my car and take her to the hospital emergency. The doctor refused to put her into the hospital. Sandy and I had an intuition that if we took mom home, we would be heading back to the hospital right away.

We decided to stay at a nearby hotel since the hospital was over forty-five miles from my parent's house.

As fate would have it, while at the hotel my mom's condition worsened. We called an ambulance. While they were tending to my mother, my father began to throw up blood. The EMT decided that both of my parents would be transported to the hospital.

Each of my parents was being checked out by a doctor simultaneously. The nurse could not get an IV into my mom's arm. I suggested that they put a hot pack on her arm and warm the vein so it can dilate and try again. The little tip worked. As I watched mom's nurse, I remember the many times Tom's chemotherapy nurse had difficulties with Tom's veins. The tip I gave mom's nurse was one Tom's nurse had used.

After talking to my sister Lindalee and explaining that the hospital was still reluctant to admit mom, she called the hospital and told them that if they did not admit our mother, she would call a lawyer. She decided she would come in person to deal with the hospital.

Almost two hours later, after Lindalee's arrival, my mom was admitted, and my dad was released. My dad wanted to stay at the hospital, but my mom's doctor told him no. We returned to the hotel.

Saturday, October 14, 2006

My mom had a heart attack early this morning while at the hospital. She already had been transferred to a hospital in Duluth early this morning. We were not informed by the hospital of her heart attack or her transfer. We found out only after a morning call to check on her health.

I drove Sandy and my dad the hour and half drive to Duluth. Sandy threw up the entire way to the hospital. My mom was in intensive care on full life support when we arrived.

The hours spent at the hospital were an emotional roller coaster. I found it difficult to spend so much time in the hospital as everything reminded me of hours Tom and I spent at hospitals and reminded me of how much I missed him.

We were not certain if mom was going to live. I was still numb from Tom's death that I did not want to think about dealing with my mom's death too.

Monday, October 23, 2006

My mom has been in full life support for the past week and half. The doctor suspects possible brain damage. I cannot imagine my mom having brain damage. She is one of those intelligent people that seem to have an answer to any questions and is enjoyable to converse with on any subject. I missed her already and did not even know her prognosis.

There were many times when I just wanted to leave the hospital. The intensive care, doctors, treatments, and the hospital itself was overwhelming. I did not want to be there, but my dad and family needed me. I have firsthand knowledge on how important family support is to recovery.

Mom's health was a distraction from Al's alcohol problems. When I finally checked in with him, he told me he was doing well. He is managing sobriety without entering a rehabilitation center.

Sunday, October 29, 2006

Mom woke from her sixteen-day coma. She did, as I had feared, show signs of brain damage. To what extent we did not know. She knew my dad right away, but she did not recognize anyone else. She was unable to walk, feed herself or pass her urine.

After two more days in intensive care, she was transferred to another floor. She will require extensive rehabilitation of which this hospital could not provide.

Wednesday, November 8, 2006

We transferred my mother to a nursing home in Spooner for rehabilitation. When my mom first arrived at the nursing home, I doubted that she would make much of a recovery. I spent almost every day at the nursing home with her. My aunt, Sue, works at the nursing home. Sue's presence gave assurance that mom would receive good care.

Sandy and I were instrumental in mom's care. My experiences in caring for Tom proved to be valuable in caring for my mother. Sandy and I hovered over our mother like hens over a chick. My mom refused to go to Physical Therapy or any of her therapies when a family member was not present, so I did spend many hours by her side.

My dad was experiencing concern, stress, and fatigue from his daily round trips of eighty miles to visit my mom over the months. Then One day, while we were visiting my mom, my dad had a mild heart attack. The impact on my mother was so great, that she was able to go to the bathroom on her own of which she had been unable to do since the heart attack. It seems that she was so concerned about my dad, that she concluded she needed to recover so she could take care of him. Her recovery progressed rapidly after this.

Sunday, November 19, 2006

Sandy and Larry moved out of my house today. They got their own apartment. I know I will miss Sandy, but I know that they could not stay forever.

Tom's Headstone
Thursday, November 23, 2006

We spent Thanksgiving at the hospital with my mom. My reflections on this Thanksgiving centered on that fact that my mom was still alive. The primary gratitude I felt was for my three children. After visiting with my mom, I drove to Gordon to visit the cemetery.

Tom's headstone had been placed and this was the first time I saw it. Tom's brother Dave paid much of the cost of the headstone. His kindness touched my heart. The headstone turned out much nicer than I had imagined. Both my and Tom's names and birth dates appeared on the stone. Tom's had a death date. It was strange to see Tom's name and a death date on the stone. It was a reality that he was dead, and I was alive.

Dream
Thursday, November 30, 2006

"Dear Tom, Last night I had a wonderful dream about you. I dreamt we were holding each other. We were together once more. It felt so good. I could touch and smell you. I carried that positive feeling with me throughout the day. Love you, Rita"

Tuesday, December 12, 2006

"Dear Tom, I had my last anal ultrasound today. I am Two years cancer free. I miss you. I am trying to go on, but it seems pointless without you. I am trying. I love you! Rita"

Opening Up To Emotional Healing
Monday, December 25, 2006

December passed quickly with many hours spent at the nursing home, which glistened with Christmas holiday decorations and activities. I had no interest in decorating my own house or even celebrating Christmas. It seemed so empty without Tom.

It turned out that my mom got a one-day leave from rehabilitation and we decided to celebrate Christmas at my house, which made the idea of decorating for Christmas more appealing. I was doing it for my mom. I wanted her and my dad to have a memorable Christmas. I was able to put my heart into decorating and cooking.

It was good to see her enjoy Christmas with her children and grandchildren surrounding her. It warmed my heart and reminded me that this is what life is all about. Enjoying and appreciated the other people in my life and not concentrating on the person I have lost.

Monday, January 1, 2007

"Tom, I really missed you last night. I became very angry because you are dead. I still feel it is so unfair. I guess that is selfish since you are the one that was cheated.

Why are you gone? What am I going to do? I have no passion or goal. I do not know where to begin. I have been wasting my time and I think you would be ashamed of me. I know I am. It has been eight months, which is very hard to believe. I wish you were here.

I wish I could talk to you and ask you what I should do with my life. I am lonely and alone. Love, Rita"

Even though I still miss Tom with my whole heart and soul, I realized that I do not cry every time I think of him. Time does help heal sorrow. There were times when I could look at a picture of him and smile from the sweet memories the picture instilled. I do not miss him any less, but I am slowly accepting that he is gone.

One day as I was sitting by my mother in the nursing home, a nurse asked me how long it had been since my husband died. Suddenly, my mom blurted out, "Tom died?"

I was surprised that she had not comprehended that Tom died. I imagine parts of her memory were damage during the heart attack. I explained to her how and when he died. She started to cry. Her tears reinforced my sense of loss.

I do not like my life without Tom because it seems meaningless and has no purpose. I try every day to find purpose. In hindsight, I realized my present purpose was to support my parents during my mother's recovery. Grief seems to block the obvious.

My energy level was low, and I was behind on my bills, which seemed complicated and frustrating. I was living on a small life insurance policy from Tom's employment and knew it would run out soon. I felt discouraged about my Social Security Disability and feared I would not get it. I feared that no one would hire me because of my osteoporosis and my combined bladder and bowel problems.

Wednesday, January 10, 2007

I yearned for a value or purpose to my life. It is difficult for me to pick up the pieces of my life and rearrange them to fit. A ray of hope did entered my life. My Social Security Disability approval came through and I will begin receiving checks in February. It is good timing as my funds are about gone.

Monday, January 15, 2007

"Tom, I am beginning to learn to be alone. It was difficult at first because I was so lonely for you. Our sweet Rascal pup is getting old. His hearing is bad, his teeth are missing, and he is losing his sight, but the little sweetheart does keep me company.

I still miss you and wish you were here, every day. I guess I am finally learning to accept that you are gone. We finally got some snow. It has not snowed all winter. It is very poor ice fishing, thin ice. You world be disappointed. Love you, Rita"

Tuesday, February 6, 2007

My mother continued with her recovery. She was released from the nursing home today and was anxious to go home. Her recover thus far is remarkable. She is a little weak with her walking but manages with a cane. She has learned to feed herself, walk again and can even write. My mom had always taken great pride in her penmanship. It is indeed a miracle of its own that she survived her heart attack and made such an amazing recovery.

She still shows signs of brain damage, but her doctor seemed to feel that her mind was so intelligent and advanced at the time of her heart attack, that it was a contributing factor to her recovery.

I know my parents will still need support and help from me in the future. I can accept tasks, not as a distraction, but as part of my life. If I remain available to offer them help, I will continue to do so.

Wednesday, February 14, 2006

Larry gave Sandy a Valentine's card and a box of chocolates. Then he turned to me and handed me a card and a box of chocolates.

He said, "I know Tom would have wanted me to give these to you, so you know that you are loved."

This simple gesture brought joy to my heart.

Friday, February 16, 2007

I began to make amazing discoveries about my abilities and myself. My truck was not starting on its own, so I took the initiative and jump-started it myself. I then plowed the driveway. Tom had taught me how to do both things before he died. It was not much, but it did give me a feeling of growth toward my independence.

February 23, 2007

I had another dream about Tom last night. We were driving to Hudson; Tom was doing the driving.

I asked him. "You don't remember me, do you?"

Tom replied, "No not really."

I said, "That's OK because you died."

Even though I do not understand the dream, I liked dreaming about Tom. I read that Edgar Cayce believed that if you dreamt about someone, it was a memory of them. I you dreamt about them and had a conversation with them, it was their spirit visiting you. I like to believe this.

Phillip and I continue to make improvements on the house. The many little things that Tom used to take care of are now my responsibility. I am developing a greater sense of confidence as I undertake more tasks around the house. I think of how many things I learned from Tom, and I am grateful that he taught me. I can handle small carpentry tasks and simple repairs. Phillip takes care of the rest. When the day arrives for

Phillip to move out, I will miss him very much. He has been my friend and companion since his father died.

I still do not yet feel independent, just existing out of necessity.

My past ideas of suicide over the past months have subsided. As the pain of Tom's loss eases, the less frequently I think about suicide. The thought of how deeply my death would hurt my children has kept me from doing it. In addition, I remember how hard Tom fought to live. How could I disgrace his memory by ending my life? Loneliness takes its toll on you. After spending so many years with the same person, it is difficult to learn how to think of me and my needs and wants. My life was wrapped up in a life that was planning and hoping for two.

Rachel and Valerie are both in Hawaii. They want me to visit. I know that I cannot handle the plane trip. My hips and legs hurt so much, and I cannot sit for that length of time. I spoke with my doctor and got a pain medication just in case I decide to go for that visit. I am depressed about having to travel alone.

Grief Support Group
March 2007

I started attending a Grief Support Group. The meetings have already been beneficial. Sharing your loss with others who have also lost a loved one, creates a strong sense of kinships and friends. I wish I had sought out a support group much sooner.

It is a place where you can share your sadness and grief without any judgement from others. It offers exercises and tasks to help you work through your grief.

Friday, March 23, 2007

"Dear Tom, I missed you today. It would have been your 53rd birthday. It felt strange not to decorate or put out balloons. I did light a candle for you. I will continue to grow old without you. I will age and you will not. It is hard to love someone so much and with so much of yourself, that when they die, much of you dies with them.

Almost a year has gone by and I still do not know what to

do with my life any more than I did right after you died. I know you would want me to be happy. My task it to find out what that is. Happy birthday and I love you. Rita"

I realized that as time passes, the pain of Tom's loss does not hurt as much as it once did. Some days it feels like yesterday. I am beginning to have more "better" days and find that I cry only a few times a week. Strange things set me off. Walking into our shop building where we spent so many hours working on cars is very difficult. The un-restored cars just sit there, and I realize they will never be finished. I just stand there and cry.

My mothers' continued recovery brings me comfort. My dad loves her as much as I loved Tom, maybe more. They have been together for over fifty-five years. I cannot imagine his loss if she had died.

Sunday, April 8, 2007

I spent Easter at my parent's house. It was also my mom's 73rd birthday. Tom's mom and brother, Al, joined us. It was nice to have all of them together at the same table. It made it easier for me to enjoy the holiday.

One-Year Anniversary
Wednesday, April 25, 2007

"Dear Tom, Yes, it has been a year and seems pretty surreal. I still cannot believe you are gone forever. Time passes. It is amazing how that happens. It passes and you remain gone. Life is still empty for me. I try to fill it up by keeping busy. The past few days I believe I have been experiencing your pain. I have been experiencing sharp, intense pain along my forehead, difficulty breathing, lower back pain and bad intestinal cramps.

A year ago, your care was intense. It was the beginning of the end. I no longer know how I feel. I have been trying to give myself permission to live. I have been trying to convince myself that it is OK to continue to live even though you have died.

It is hard to explain. Our lives were so dependent upon each other for companionship, dreams, and challenges. We were each other's accomplishments, happiness, and purpose for living.

It is awfully hard to fill all those roles when I am alone. Being alone is extremely hard after thirty years of always having someone. Is it OK if I go on living? I know your main purpose in life was for me to be happy. Right now, I don't think I will ever be happy again. I need to feel right about continuing to live. I need permission. I need to know it is OK. I need to know that it isn't selfish to continue without you.

Do you understand what I am saying? Does it make sense to you? I know what you asked for before you died. I have done some of those things and I am working on the rest.

For now, I still hate to think of my future, and I know one day that I will have to think about it. I love and miss you. Rita"

I never thought I would be able to say this but thinking of Tom at this time is not as painful as it had been. I am trying to grasp being alive. As a cancer survivor, I should already have a good concept of what it is like to survive death. Missing Tom has made it difficult to celebrate this wonderful accomplishment.

The Grief Support Group meetings are going quite well. We shared pictures of our loved ones and shared what they meant to us. I brought our wedding picture and all of Toms' fishing pictures. I know everyone else at the group feels their loss as greatly as I feel mine. Losing someone you love, hurts, no matter what the relationship was.

I have been transcribing my journal notes, so they are all together. The journal entries are full of reminders and created a heavy, tight pain in my chest.

Sunday, April 29, 2007

"Dear Tom, I saw a deer this morning. The weather is finally getting nice. I am not sure, but I think this entry is to say "Goodbye". It is one year that you have been dead. I think it feels like I am not moving on. I do not want to move on, but I am sure you would want me to. I miss you so much. It still hurts. I can hardly breathe it hurts so much. So alone and I do not like it at all.

What am I going to do with the rest of my life? You are not a part of it. It was supposed to be that way, but it is not. It does not make sense what has happened and all that is still happening. I need something in my life.

I love you and miss you. I wish you were not dead. I wish you were here, and I wish you could come back. I know you cannot, and I know you never will. I love you! Rita"

I realize that I am at peace with not killing myself. I remember a movie I saw and where someone said, "People who kill themselves go to another place." I do not want to take the chance that I would ruin all chances of ever being reunited with Tom again.

I know that Tom would be heart broke and disappointed with me if I were to kill myself. I am OK with it now. I know that everyone who losses someone they love will feel overwhelming pain. It hurts more than anything will ever hurt. I am trying to live again. It is still going to take time.

Thursday, May 10, 2007

"Dear Tom, I decided that I want to keep writing to you. It helps me not miss you so much. Silly, I guess.

Today is my birthday. I am sitting here crying. I can hardly see through my tears. I am remembering the day Dr. H. told us you only had nine to twelve months to live. When he told us, you were terminal. The support group went well.

I cried a lot there too. Combined with all the crying I did today, I guess the value of the support group help to release the pressure I had been feeling. Love and miss you, Rita."

I thought about the reasons why I feel so lost. I am facing life by myself for the first time as a disabled person. I was not disabled before my cancer. I was not a widow before my cancer. I had a life before both of our cancers and now I have a new one. It is different because Tom died, and I am a disabled widow.

I have to find the new person I am because of my cancer and because of Toms' death. I need to deal with my physical limitations and my emotional needs. I am physically tired and emotionally drained from cancer and grief.

Do I feel this sense of lost because of my physical limitations? Do I feel this loss because Tom died? Do I feel lost because my parents need more help and support because of mom's health?

I have so many changes and adjustments going on all at once. I cannot differentiate which situation is causing what emotions. I feel overwhelmed with too many emotions from too many sources. It seems the emotions are mostly negative. My goal is to sort out which emotions result from what situation and apply a tactic to create a more positive response.

Saturday, May 12, 2007

Rachel's boyfriend Bart spent the day with me. He was helping with some light yard work. I really like him and so did Tom. Bart pleasantly surprised me.

We were sitting outside eating lunch when he said he has something to ask me.

"I would like to ask you if it is alright with you if I marry Rachel?"

His sentiment touched my soul. Asking for a daughters' hand in marriage was so quaintly old fashion. His request brought me to joyful tears. Of course, I said yes. He was going to join Rachel in Hawaii for a brief vacation and planned to propose to her while he was there. Then he and Rachel would fly back home to Wisconsin together. It was so exciting.

Saturday, May 19, 2007

"Dear Tom, twenty-eight years ago we began our life together as husband and wife. Well, we made it, "Until Death do us Part". That is the only thing that would have separated us. I still love you so much. Even though your physical being is gone, I am still in love with you. I cherish all the wonderful memoires we created together and the fabulous children we created.

Rachel and Bart are engaged. How wonderful. Our little girl is getting married. Bart is a good man and I cannot think of anyone else who will cherish her and treat her better than him. They are both lucky to have found each other.

Happy Anniversary! We had a very good life together. I love you. Rita"

Upon reflection, I realized that this was the last time I wrote "Dear Tom" at the beginning of my journal entry. Subconsciously I was ready to move on with my life.

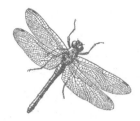

CHAPTER 16 - RECOVERY AS A CANCER SURVIVOR AND WIDOW

July 2007

My recent appointment with Dr. H. went well. Both my blood count and my chest x-rays were good. I will be having another colonoscopy in August. I had some blood in my stools and he wants to check to make sure it is not anything serious. He thinks it is just radiation-damaged tissue.

I am afraid to have cancer again. I have been having bloody stools, but it is different than it had been before my diagnosis.

My thoughts about living are becoming more and more positive each day. Rachel's upcoming wedding is a positive inspiration. They are beginning a life together and I feel great joy for them both.

The wedding plans are keeping me busy, only this time the busyness is for me. It is for my daughter and for me. It feels good to do something positive and interesting. I do wish Tom were here for her wedding, but I know he will be here in spirit.

My heart was joyously filled when my nieces, nephews, and children all showed up one weekend to clean, repair and prep the yard and house for the wedding reception. Brush was cut and moved, dead trees cut down, trash all collected and disposed of and a lot of visiting. It was a positive day and seemed like old times when our family used to get together for all the holidays and birthdays.

When they finished, everything looked perfect.

Thursday, August 2, 2007

For the wedding reception, we went with a Hawaiian theme since Rachel and Bart were engaged in Hawaii. The tent, tables, chairs, and porta-potties arrived. Jessie and I hung lights around the inside of the tent, and it looked very festive. Sandy and I made a volcano out of plaster of Paris and used a small humidifier that had a red, smoky light to create a smoky volcano look.

Rachel's Wedding and the Butterfly

Friday, August 3, 2007

The wedding ceremony was Friday night as Bart's family home. The ceremony took place by the river near their house. Tom's brothers and my family all attended except Tom's mother. She was in the hospital.

During the vows, a black butterfly sat on the ground at Rachel's feet. It then flew in and out of the chairs where the guests sat. As we moved up the hill to the fabulous meal Bart's mother had prepared, the butterfly came with us. Larry took me aside and said, "That butterfly is Tom. He told me he borrowed the butterfly's body for the wedding". I believed him.

It seems as though many other people felt the same about the butterfly but did not say anything until later when we were sharing pictures, some of which included the butterfly.

Saturday, August 4, 2007

Since the reception was a Hawaiian theme, everyone was dressed in Hawaiian dresses and shirts. I kept Tom's collection of Hawaiian shirts because of my emotional attachment to them. I invited anyone who did not have his or her own Hawaiian shirt to borrow one of Tom's.

The wedding reception was a great party. All the relatives who attend the wedding also came to the reception. Many friends came as well. It was a potluck reception with a hitch. Whatever dish a person brought to pass, had to include a recipe card. These cards were put into a special recipe box, which was later given to Rachel and Bart as a gift.

Tents were pitched for overnight guests and the ones without a personal tent, slept in the dinning tent. It was great fun! The festivities and uniqueness of Rachel's' wedding reminded me of how much fun my and Tom's wedding had been. I did not feel the sorrow at Rachel's wedding that I had felt at her college graduation. Strangely, a butterfly came to the reception as well. The presence of the butterfly helped me to believe that Tom was at her wedding and that created a warm place in my heart. I think it was the same one. I like to think so, anyway.

The business of the wedding preparation was uplifting. Now I feel overwhelmed with "nothingness". I can do whatever or go wherever I want, but I have nothing to do or nowhere to go.

September 2007

Rachel and Bart moved to Oregon and Val returned to her home in Hawaii. I felt the empty nest syndrome all over again. It seemed worse this time because previously I had Tom to lean on.

I spent more time with my mom and dad, but that depressed me. I hate seeing mom the way she is. Her dependency on others reminds me of Tom. She is improving all the time and that does make me happy.

I have always enjoyed writing and secretly believe it is my purpose and passion. My goal is to cultivate my writing ideas and discover my purpose in life through my writing.

Friday, September 14, 2007

I have been writing in my journal on a more regular basis since I am striving for a discovery and a new beginning for myself. I am going to review many of my past entries and use the feelings I have written down to continue with this discovery.

I sometimes wonder what is wrong with me. Why can't I go on with my life? Why I am so depressed? I dwell on the "what if" of my life instead of what it can be. I plan to analyze the negativity in my journals and convert them into either acceptance or a positive action. I revert to depressed thoughts and feelings and entertain them. I plan to stop doing this and move forward in a positive manner.

Moving Forward - Analyzing My Life
Singular personal identity - Widow

I found some difficulties analyzing my new life and who I am as a singular person. Becoming a widow is a passage from one life to another. It is becoming single when you had no choice in the matter. As a couple, much of what I wanted developed from the relationship I shared with my husband. I still feel happiness in my children's happiness, joy, and success. I feel joy in helping others.

I need to reach beyond these things to find happiness and joy within my own life. As the years have passed, I have discovered that many of the same things in my past that brought me happiness and joy, are still true, even without Tom's presence. I can bring past enjoyments into my future.

I enjoy working on jewelry, home remolding and redecorating, writing and watching great movies. I am learning to do these things to please me, to make me happy. Most of the time it is enough. As I sort through the materialistic aspects of my life, I find it is healthy for me to let go of the things that were "ours". I have kept personal keepsakes that bring me wonderful memories. I have discovered that decorating my house with items that solely reflect me have helped me to re-discover my likes and interests.

I once heard that your loved one is never really gone until they are forgotten. As I did my redecorating, I incorporated a wall that is dedicated to Tom's memory. It has the memorial plaque I received from Lindalee and Jeff, Tom's picture, a couple of duck statures. It also includes a pounded copper picture frame Rachel and Valerie created with a picture of themselves as small children. They had given it to Tom as a birthday gift on his last birthday. Last is the small blue and silver personal urn with Tom's ashes.

The little shrine helps me to remember the wonderful man I married.

Financial future

When Tom was still alive, we took care of finances together. Tom had a good income, and I made some income with internet selling. We had a budget and leisure time funds set aside. Tom was always on top of his investments. I was primarily in charge of the checking account and paying the bills.

The years during both of our cancer treatments became a great financial burden. I was unable to generate income while going through treatment and when Tom's diagnosis came about in the middle to this, financial recovery was not possible. As Tom lost some of his income and the medical bills grew, I did have worries about my financial future even before he died.

We had no life and casualty insurance on our mortgage, a big oversight, and I knew that would become my responsibly after Tom died. He had a modest life insurance policy through work, but I did not realize it would not go very far after he died.

I have created a budget and an overall financial picture so I know what I can and cannot afford. I used much of the insurance to pay my very expensive COBRA insurance until I became eligible for Medicare.

My lifestyle has change dramatically without the nice income Tom and I had shared. I have learned to make do with only the necessities of life such as modest food purchases, secondhand clothes, and no cable. My cell phone is a bare bones contract for emergencies.

I resolve to become more knowledgeable about investments and find a stockbroker that I feel comfortable with and trust.

The medical bills still exist, and I have been able to set up payments with the bills I owe. It seems like it will take a lifetime to pay the thousands of dollars I owe from both my and Tom's treatments, but I pay each month and just accept that these will be a part of my life forever.

Letting go of Anger

I realize that I carry an excess amount of anger with me each day. I am angry because I feel cancer robbed us of quality time before Tom died. The anger is wrapped up with grief and sadness as well. When I remember Tom's home health care, I feel anger and the pain of watching him so vulnerable, helpless, and dependent. The actual care was not the painful memory but the fact that his great efforts to live were unsuccessful.

I am not angry for providing this care for Tom, I feel satisfied that Phillip and I provided the best care we could give. Through our efforts we showed Tom our love for him up until and after his death.

The question of why us, is slowly being replace with acceptance. Acceptance that Tom died, and I must go on with my life the best I can, which will allow me to live as well as I can. I will always cherish the memories and life that we shared and will love Tom forever. Tom would want me to continue with with my life as best I can.

Dealing With Grief

Part of my grief is morning the future that Tom and I had planned is now gone and accept that I have a future of my own to plan and live. I also have accepted that Tom wanted me to be happy while we were together and even though we are no longer together, it is still Tom's wish. am grieving the loss of a friend, companion, and soul mate. Loneliness is also part of my grief. I have not yet discovered how to deal with the loneliness, but I have faith that time will present some answers for me.

Once again acceptance is the best way to deal with another aspect of my grief and healing.

Fears of cancer returning and dealing with disability

I fear that my cancer will return. It may be that once you have had cancer, fear of it returning, is a greater than the fear that you may develop cancer. I know that if I eat well, take care of my present health issues and follow a exercise program, I am doing all that I can to prevent it from returning. I have had to teach myself not to worry if it may return and realized that I will have to deal with it if it does return. In other words, not to create heartache and grief over something that may never happen.

I still experience frustration and tears relating to my physical limitations. It is the remembering my lost abilities that cause me so much frustration. To deal with these emotions, I remind myself of the things I can do and the degree of independence I still have.

Bladder control pads give me the ability to leave the house and go places such as shopping, movies or out with family or friends. A cane helps reduce the repeated hip and leg fatigue I experience when walking, allowing me to be mobile without a wheelchair.

My anger about my limitations is becoming less and less as I learn to deal with my limitations. Once again, anger is being replaced with acceptance.

A Place Called Home

I have fears that I will not be able to remain in my home. My house is my comfort zone. I feel secure about where I live but fear that financially I may lose my house. I enjoy living in the country with all the trees and the animals that stop by and visit. I find it almost impossible to think about town or city living. It makes me feel closed in.

For now, I can make the mortgage and property taxes based on my income. Over the past few years, repairs and maintenance have eaten much of my savings. This is where my fear comes in. What will I do when I can no longer afford repairs and maintenance?

Again, I need to put these fears aside and not worry about what may or may not happen. I need to take joy in the fact that I still live in my home. I need to realize that when I have to make a decision about living elsewhere, I will be able to deal with it if the time comes. I want to be able to smile with sincerity and remind myself that life is worth living, no matter what.

There are many discoveries ahead of me if I can put all the

fears about my future aside and be positive.

My fears are my insecurities about my life. I am adjusting to being alone in many areas of my life. I do have my children and family of which I am grateful. My healing must begin with giving myself permission to live. Not let my fears of the past and non-existent fears of the future to pave the way for my life.

Some of the fear of being alone also involves making decisions alone. I need to have enough faith in myself to trust that I will make the right decisions in my life.

After Tom's death I was fearful of what to do with my life. To camouflage this fear, I become completely involved in the problems and dealings of my family. It was a substitute for or to avoid creating a new life of my own. As my fear of what to do with my life becomes less prominent, I am learning to say no when others make requests of me for things I do not want to do. I no longer need to substitute their lives for mine.

Learn to value myself

Throughout my marriage, Tom's approval of my accomplished fueled me to go on. His approval no longer exists so I am left with giving myself this approval and realized my accomplishments for myself. I need to realize that I am important and that I have the right to continue with my life.

I must also realize that I do have something to offer others as long as I set boundaries, so my needs come first. I can do volunteer work for both personal satisfaction and the value of helping others. It would also serve to get me out of the house and interact with other people.

The guilt I felt that I survived. I often thought that it was me that should have died because Tom had so much more to offer our children and the world. I believed that his life had more value than mine. I now realized that each of us has our own value in life. That no one person has more value than another. We each contribute what we have and if it is our best, the value is immeasurable, no matter who you are and what you have contributed.

Many years ago, I was a weekly columnist and freelance reporter. I remember the great pleasure I obtained through my writing. The writer within me has been dormant these past years. As I began writing what would become an extremely emotional book, slowly the writer re-appeared.

For many years, one definition of success for me is to become a published writer. If I want to become a successful writer, I can be one. I control it. I decide it. It is my choice. My many past newspaper publications already defines that I am a successful writer. The next step is to create a book worthy of publication. This is one of my life's goals. Re-connecting to the writer within me, is reconnecting with a part of me from my past and means learning about the new person I am becoming.

Monday, September 17, 2007

At one point in time, Tom had foot casts made for corrective insoles for his shoes. I found them today and decided to put the foot casts under the memorial apple tree. I wished him a good journey. I really miss him and still cannot believe or understand why he had to die. I realize that I do not cry as often as I used to, even though I felt at one time that the pain would last forever. I do not love Tom any less, but I am learning to love him in a different way.

I love him through positive memories and find comfort that I am accepting the idea that I can learn to live without him. Not just being alive, but also actually learning to live. It is not an easy task but through some mystery I cannot define, it does get easier as time goes by.

Friday, September 21, 2007

I realized a big change that I have made. I stopped writing my journal to Tom. I think it indicates that I am accepting that he is gone. While I wrote to him, it was as if he was only away, not gone. I still cannot believe that he is dead and still cannot understand why.

Reality is very difficult to accept when it is so painful. I wish Tom were here more than anything else in my life. Time passes, the sun rises and sets, and I am still here. Life continues and what I do with it becomes not only my legacy, but Tom's as well.

Tuesday, September 25, 2007

I was adventurous today. I met Lindalee and Jeff at the casino to watch the Packer/Viking game on the big screens. I really enjoyed watching the game with other people. It was great fun! I felt happy and enjoyed it.

Tom's Presence
Friday, October 19, 2007

I have been feeling sad the past few days. This morning as I walked into the kitchen, I felt a peace or warmth pass over me. I was standing in the same area of the kitchen where I stood after Tom died when I felt as though Tom was hugging me. I guess he gave me another hug this morning. I felt something "special" to ease the sadness. I believe it was he and it made me feel happy.

I continue to be of help to my parents even though the long drive up north tires me. I understand how difficult it is to raise children while making sacrifices as parents along the way. As their children, we have the opportunity to repay them. I am comfortable with helping my parents out as long as I am able. It is a rewarding experience knowing that my parents understand that they are loved.

Tuesday, October 23, 2007

Sandy and Larry moved back into my house. With Larry's multiple surgeries from back injuries, they could not afford their apartment anymore. It has only been one year since they moved out.

Thursday, November 1, 2007

Phillip and Jessie moved out. I hated to see Phillip leave. I knew it would happen eventually but having him here gave me a sense of security. It helped me not to miss Tom so much.

Monday, November 5, 2007

My little dog, Rascal is getting old. I enjoy his companionship. He seems to be a link between Tom and me. I faced the need to take him to the vet. My desire to keep him longer blurred the fact that it was his time. He cannot see or hear and chokes on his food, even if I soften it. I will miss him. The vet was kind and understanding and made Rascal's passing as painless as possible. They made a cast paw print and I placed it by Tom's memorial picture.

The maintenance of the house is overwhelming. I am not used to taking care of everything myself. It is a difficult adjustment. It is strange to have to pay people to fix things because I am used to Tom fixing them.

I know I am much stronger than I have been acting. I can do it on my own; I just have to believe in myself. I have to realize I can have a life without Tom. It is not something I ever planned for, but the reality is that he is gone and I am on my own. I have to make the best of it.

Sunday, December 30, 2007

My septic system has backed again. It is the second time in three days and the fourth time over the past several months. The care of the septic was not one of my chores, but now it is. It seems the pipe between the solid holding tank and the liquid tank collapsed. It will have to be dug up in the spring and the pipe replace. It is augured out for now and should hold up until then.

January 2008

My new year includes streamlining my house. I have decided to eliminate as many unnecessary items as I can. I guess a good cleaning out will help to lose a lot of excess emotional baggage as well. Paperwork and memorabilia are difficult to sort. Some items of my and Tom's past conjure up many memories. Sometimes I cry and sometimes I do not. Many memories are positive, but the realization that Tom is gone causes chest tightness and tears. I analyze each item and decide if it is worth keeping.

My theory is to do it one time through, wait a short period of time and do it again. I am hoping I can release the emotional attachment I may have assign an item when I go through it a second time.

When I think about creating a positive life for myself, I begin to fear that my cancer will come back. It seems like I am destined to live of life of woe. It is my punishment? Punishment for what I am not sure. Maybe this fear is part of the reason I am afraid to accept being alive without Tom.

Thursday, January 17, 2008

I am having another colonoscopy and I once again dread the preparation for it. I know I can do this. The preparation for colostomy had changed for the better. This time I had two doses of a pill to take and less than half of the liquid to drink. The liquid laxative has also improved in taste. It is still difficult to prepare for, but as I struggled through the doses of preparation, I told myself it is for me, my children and for Tom. When I get negative results from the test, I know I will be ready to start a new life.

Thursday, January 24, 2008

I have been enjoying making jewelry the last two days. I am using new combinations of materials and I am enjoying the result. My daughter Val gave me a great perk today. She told me she was grateful that Tom and I gave her life. I am also grateful for that. She also told me that she wanted me to find myself. I am working on that.

Right now, I feel positive about life and that I do have a future. Then later, I feel sad and lost again. I hate these strange mood swings. They seem too complicated.

Wednesday, January 29, 2008

I do not think God chooses who lives or who dies. I had been taught that God gave man the freedom of choice and that God does not control our lives. If this is true, then God would not choose who would live or die, because if He did, He would be controlling our lives.

I believe God gives abilities as gifts to the healers of our world whether they are natural healers or medical healers. The healers' skills, the person's own strength to live and health advancements are what help people to live.

My mom survived because of the care she received and her own physical and mental ability to live. Tom's body became so damaged from treatments and the cancer growth that his body could not go on. I cannot blame God for Tom's death.

I have not prayed since Tom died. I know that prayer makes us think positively. Prayer gives us strength because we believe things will be better. Once we believe wholly, things are better. Positive thinking gives positive results while negative thinking gives negative results.

Looking for the good in our lives will at least result in a positive attitude. Dwelling on the negative creates sadness and depression.

I am going to concentrate on looking at the good in this world. I need to open my eyes. Being alive each day is good. I realize that bad things are going to happen around us each day, but I need to filter them out. I need to see past the bad and look for the good.

A warm sunny day is good. Being alive and able to see a blizzard or feel the sub-zero weather means I am alive. Being alive is good.

When I feel lonely, it tells me I need a positive change. It tells me I am alive and want something more in my life. To heal my loneliness does not mean I need another man in my life, just other people. I spent much of my time in my house. I can cure this situation through volunteer work. It is a good place to start.

Being a part of something can heal loneliness. The grief group helped while it lasted. I miss the group and need to find another source to be a part of something. The positives in my life are that I have a house to live in, I am cancer free, and I have some form of income. I am skilled and talented, which gives me the opportunity to be better than I am today and feel accomplished. It is these traits will help me to succeed.

I can give my sister and her husband a place to live, a refuge for a while. I can be helpful to my parents and my children when they call me for advice, which makes me feel useful.

I think we tend to beat ourselves up with negative think-

ing. We think we have to define our lives as "something" to justify our existence. We are not happy with just being alive. Our
happiness, peace and sense of who we are, come from within.
We become so caught up with defining the reason for being, that
we forget to "just be". We burden ourselves with the tasks of
defining ourselves that we forget to live. Accepting that we are
alive and that it is good enough is our choice.

It is my choice, not Tom's death, not my disability and not
my loneliness. It is me, all me, that makes the choice. I can no
longer continue with "What would Tom want?" I know what he
wanted, but he is gone. I can no longer live just waiting to define
my life. I want to be able to control my own life. I make the good
and bad decisions now. If I am to survive, it will be by my own
merits.

I have this feeling of almost making it. It is the point
where I can go on living positively and not negatively. I cannot
explain the feeling. Maybe it is anticipation, or it is permission
to live beyond Tom. I want my life to mean something for me
and to have a purpose for me. I want to find my own form of
peace.

Wednesday, March 4, 2008

I am dealing with another bladder infection and once
again I am on an antibiotic. I truly hope that they will not be a
permanent part of my life.

Sunday, March 23, 2008

Today would have been Tom's 54th birthday. I lit a candle
for him.

Two-Year Anniversary
Tuesday, April 25, 2008

It has been two years now and I still miss Tom. It is
strange that he died on a Tuesday and today is also a Tuesday. I
still have difficulty realizing that it is true. Sandy and Larry are
still living with me. While they are living here, I am finding it a
struggle to define my own independence. So much of their life
blends into mine. They are a couple and strive to develop their

future as a couple.

I have a strong need to discover myself. My parents taught us to care for our family whenever we can. Since they have nowhere else to go, they will be here for a while longer. My need to be on my own is great and I hope I can continue with my growth even with them still living here. It is impossible to think that their difficulties will not affect me because it does. We are working things out so all of us can continue living in the same house. It is nice to have Sandy's company.

I still push myself physically. I still have difficulty accepting my limitations and become frustrated with them.

I still deal with the pangs of "what if" when I think about Tom. I know this is negative thinking, so I try to replace these thoughts with more positive ones. Thinking about my children and their lives does help. They are all doing well, and this makes me happy.

I am happy with my decision to stay on my land. I enjoy it here and it brings me peace. I know I can find a way to make it work. I am taking it a day at a time and not creating problems before they arise. Each day of peace is another day toward my happiness.

July 2008

Once again, my time is filled with care of my family. Larry has had two more back surgeries since they moved back into my house. I have been being supportive of both he and Sandy.

My dad had three hernia surgeries in the past two months. After each surgery, he and my mother come to my house for recovery. It is easier for me to care for them at my house then at theirs. I do not mind offering my care to them. I love them and want to be make positive contributions to their lives. I am available to help them, and it feels like a good thing to do.

I miss seeing my daughters. Valerie moved from Hawaii to Oregon last December of where Rachel and Bart moved to shortly after their wedding. Both of my daughters want me to come for a visit. As soon as there are no more surgeries in my families' future, I want to be daring and take a road trip to

Oregon. I am looking forward to an adventure. In my younger years, when I lived in Montana, I used to drive between Montana and Wisconsin in one day. I know I cannot endure that type of a trip, so I am going to take my time getting there and utilize a thing called a hotel.

My Freedom Road Trip
Thursday, August 7 – 29, 2008

I am proud of myself. I drove to Portland, OR and visited with my daughters. I took my time and stayed in hotels along the way. I made sure I ate right and did not tire myself out. It took a little longer, but I did it.

It was enjoyable to visit with my children. I got to know Val's boyfriend, Eduardo much better and had fun just hanging out with them.

On my way back to Wisconsin, I stopped in Columbia Falls, Montana to visit my aunt Billie, my uncle Merle and my cousins. I lived there over thirty years ago and had not been back since I moved. It is amazing how things change.

Taking a trip like this on my own gave me a feeling of accomplishment. I have developed a greater appreciation of my abilities.

September 2008

I continue to struggle with repeated bladder infections. I seem to get one every other month. It bothers me to have to take antibiotics all the time. I have tried cranberry juice and dried cranberries to ward off the infections, but it does not seem to help. I need to do more research to find something that will help.

I started counseling again today. I felt that maybe another person's insight into my life might help me get a new perspective of the direction I should go. I stopped taking an antidepressant a few months ago. I like who I am without it. Self-help books and nutritional supplements such as St. Johns Wart seem to be helping.

If I find myself slipping into a chronic depression, I will reconsider going on an antidepressant again.

Larry had another surgery. His diabetes is taking it toll on his body. It is a good thing that I can offer support to both Sandy and Larry during their time of need. It helps me to repay the support they offered to Tom and I during my cancer treatments. It is a good thing.

Thursday, September 25, 2008

I have been taking flowers to Tom's grave every six months. I make the silk arrangements, so they include red roses and yellow daffodils. The red roses are for love and the yellow daffodils for in memory of his fight against cancer. I still feel a great loss when I go to the cemetery. It is strange, but I do not talk to Tom while I am at the cemetery. I pet the stone and leave the flowers, but I do not talk. However, I frequently talk to him within my mind. I feel more of a connection to him within myself than through something external.

When I was visiting with my mother the other day, she said she could see the sadness in my eyes. I can too. I know the sadness of Tom's loss looms within me. I realized that many people think I should be over my grieving, fully accept that Tom is gone, and go on with my life.

It does not bother me. I am not on anyone's time line to be done with my morning. I feel justified in taking my own time. After all, how can I rush such an emotion? I do not cry as much I have in the past months. I am able to think about Tom and smile. I can look at his pictures and remember the good things we had and not feel regret.

Cancer in the Family

Tuesday, October 14, 2008

Once again, cancer has touched my family. My sister Lindalee's daughter, Diana received a diagnosis of thyroid cancer. She is finding her own way to deal with it. I know her future is going to be full of changes and adjustments compiled with many emotions. I hope she feels enough trust in me to confide in if she feels a need.

Zometa - Osteoporosis
Thursday, October 16, 2008

I had another bone density test this week. There is no improvement and some worsening in the osteoporosis of my hips and pelvis. The Fosamax was not beneficial. At my appointment today, Dr. H. and I disguised my hip and pelvic pain combined with the osteoporosis. Dr. H. decided to try Zometa. Zometa is a very potent intravenous bisphosphonate used to reduce bone pain and helps restore the normal process of bone remodeling, thus reducing the chance of bone complications such as bone fracture.

Zometa is beneficial to patients who already have Osteoporosis, which affects millions of postmenopausal women in the United States. In addition to the Zometa, I am taking supplements such as calcium intake (at least 1200 mg daily for postmenopausal women) and a vitamin D (400 to 800 IU daily) and do regular weight bearing exercise. I do not drink but I do have an urgent need to stop smoking since smoking is the worst thing to be doing with osteoporosis.

Prior to my IV, I had a blood test done to make sure my kidneys are functioning normally. My creatine was checked, and I am just inside the safe zone for the IV. I will receive Zometa through an IV two times per year, every six months. I am hopeful that my radiated bones will benefit from this treatment.

Tuesday, October 28, 2008

It has only been two weeks since Diana's news about cancer when we received yet another shock. My sister Val's daughter, Christina, also received a diagnosis of thyroid cancer. What are the odds of them both discovery their cancer only weeks apart and the same cancer?

I hate the sound of that. I fear for both of them. I know how devastating cancer can be on your life and I hope with my whole heart that they have an easier time than I did.

Friday, November 7, 2008

Since I am concentrating on the good things in life, my

revelation for the day is I am important to my children and that makes me feel important in my life.

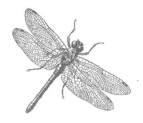

CHAPTER 17 - RECOVERY CONTINUES

Saturday, November 22, 2008

Journal entry: Trenches of Sorrow

"I have crossed over the trenches of total sorrow. The murky waters no longer have their hold on me, sucking me downward. The heavy pressure upon my body has relinquished, enabling me to rise to the surface.

Memories of my journey through sorrow still linger, but no longer pull me downward. I have reached the banks on the other side of sorrow. Now I must pull myself upon the shores of healing and strength and learn to live beyond sadness and pain.

The shore is the gateway to my new future. The new journey will continue to have its trials but as I climb upon the shore, I will not be alone. On the other side, I will find a companion. That companion is hope."

By Rita K. Kasinskas

Tom's Quilts
Tuesday, December 16, 2008

I finally did something I had said I would do. I made personal quilts for my children. I still had Tom's Hawaiian shirts plus his T-shirts, chambray shirts and his housecoats.

I am not a quilter but decided that simple would be OK. I cut all the shirts and housecoats into squares and sorted them. The quilts are personal sized. I created simple patterns for each quilt and sewed them together. I put these squares on a twin-sized blanket and stitched along each square to bind the top and bottom together. I think they turned out quite well.

Sandy and Larry went to Oregon to visit their children and grandchildren. They delivered the two quilts to Rachel and Valerie. The girls instantly recognized some of the shirts. Phillip was pleased to receive his quilt as well. Giving them some warm memories of their father seemed best done this way.

My children told me the quilts were one of the best gifts they had ever received. For the rest of the family, I took the reaming scraps from Tom's clothes and covered plain, round, Christmas ornaments. The results had a quilted look. I will give the ornaments as gifts when we get together for Christmas dinner at Lindalee's house.

Further Emotional Growth
Monday, December 22, 2008

I have discovered that I let weeks go by before I leave the house. I tell myself I am too tired, or I have nowhere to go. Secretly I think I am hiding from life. I am losing my contact with people. Even though I do not have a job, I can go grocery shopping at least once per week. I made a pact with myself to visit mom and dad at least twice a month.

Thinking positive and presenting myself in a positive manner will help me to live positive.

Thursday, December 25, 2008

I spent Christmas Eve alone since the family get together was not planned until Saturday. Being alone was not as bad as I thought it would be. I missed Tom and my children, though. Each year I write Tom a Christmas letter to let him know how the year had gone. Being alone gave me the quite time I needed. I guess the Christmas letter became my substitute for writing my journal entries to him.

Saturday, December 27, 2008

Today I am four years cancer free.

Thursday, January 1, 2009

259

I spent New Year's Eve alone. I missed the lobster dinners that Tom used to make. I miss him. I had some pizza and watched a movie. It was peaceful.

I am hopeful as I start a new year. I can create new habits, new goals, and renewed health. I will worry less and be more responsible. I will smile more and try to take a positive outlook on life. At least these things are a start. I will keep an activity log so I can see my improvements and be positive about those things.

I have accepted that Tom is gone, and I can have a good life without him. I will stop feeling guilty because there is no reason to feel guilty. I am going to believe in myself no matter what I do, which will help me to find my passion, purpose, and goal.

I accept the presence of God with my own understanding of what that means to me. I will resolve my anger and accept that the future Tom and I had planned is gone. I will accept that the future I will now plan is mine and will be worthwhile and meaningful.

I will learn to accept that for now, I am on my own, and that it may be permanent and that is OK. I will develop a social life. I will accept that my parents count on me for support. I am valuable to them, and I accept it as an honor.

I will create a ten-year financial plan and do what it takes to make it a reality.

Tuesday, January 6, 2009

I am cleaning the china hutch. There are many memories. Some are pleasant even with the pain. Things like our wedding glasses, the children's hand molds and our monogrammed wine set. Sometimes it is hard to deal with, but I am trying to accept these memoires in a positive way.

I am getting many things done while Sandy and Larry are in Oregon but making a mess as I go. I am avoiding working on Tom's book. (Tom's book is the book you are now reading.) I have a good start and it will come in its own time.

I feel I need to get house things done before Sandy and Larry return. I lose ambition to get things done when they are here. Maybe because I usually make such a mess as I go along, and I know they do not understand and do not like the mess.

I want organization so I feel like I have control over my life.

February 2009

Diana and Christina are dealing with their cancer. Christina's future is promising as they did get all the cancer. Diana has metastasized and is still undergoing treatments.

I went on Medicare this month. COBRA payments were expensive. The new coverage is scary. I am not used to having a basic medical coverage. It makes me worry about my medical future, especially if my cancer were to return. Again, as part of my personal growth, I will think positive and not allow myself to experience stress cover something that may not happen.

My Peace with Spirituality
February 23, 2009

I have been doing some thinking what I believe about God as the Almighty and religion. Belief in God is purely a spiritual experience between an individual and the Creator Himself. When you establish a relationship with someone, you do not go to a friend or relative and ask what your relationship with that person should be. You use your own sense of perception about that person and let your heart and soul guide you to the distinctive relationship you will have with them.

Over the past three years, I have been offered so many versions of where I should be in my faith with God, that I was rejecting them all. Now I have discovered my own relationship with the Almighty based on spirituality, which has given me the connection to faith that I have been seeking.

Monday, March 23, 2009

Today would have been Tom's 55th birthday. I quit smoking a few days ago.

As I think about the empowerment of my life, I realize that I do control my life. If I want it, I must achieve it. If I need it, I must obtain it. I must not feel fear to fix or obtain what is rightfully mine – no fear. No one else will or can help me obtain what

I need or want. I cannot rely on others for support so I must lean on myself. I must care about my own life.

I must be strong, brave, independent and assertive. I think life was easier for me when I had Tom to share my thoughts and ideas. I realize that I have been feeling sorry for myself and have not been moving forward with my life.

On a movie I recently saw, a women said about the death of another's' husband. "Your life begins when his life ends." I have no doubt in the truth of this. My new life began when Tom's life ended. However, it is mine and I need to start over. I feel a strength within me that has been sleeping the past three years. It was nurtured by sorrow and depression.

Saturday, April 25, 2009

It is three years now and it still seems like yesterday in many ways. I have accepted Tom's death, but I am still reluctant to give up my sorrow. I am now able to see life in a positive way, and I am hopeful about my future.

I was at a local health fair helping a hypnotist friend of mine at her booth. As I was wondering around the fair, I stopped at a past life booth. The woman at the booth said I harbored anger from a past life. I told her it was not from a past life but my present life.

"Today is the third anniversary of my husband's death. I still love him and miss him." I explained to her as I began to cry.

Before I realized what was happening, a woman was standing beside me and she said, "Excuse me for interrupting, but he is standing right behind you."

I continued crying.

The women told me that Tom loves me and visits me in my dreams at least once a month. She continued to say that Tom did not want to see me so lonely and that he is sending someone for me. She said that I should not feel guilty about it because he is picking this person especially for me, but I must wait one more year.

The tears continued to roll down my face. I then asked her why Tom always comes up behind me to give me a hug. She replied that he is pulling all the goodness from the world and wrapping me in it.

My tears become tears of happiness. I carried the positive feelings I receives with me for many days that followed.

Sunday, May 3, 2009

I have been working on the couple with cancer book. It has been emotional but healing. Reliving the events over those years has given me a new insight to my feelings and the progression through this tough journey that Tom and I took together. I have decided to take a break from it though. I have reached the part where Tom has passed and I cannot handle the emotions right now.

Wednesday, May 20, 2009

I feel very accomplished. I refinanced my mortgage at a reduced interest rate. As I signed my name on the dotted line, I thought of how proud Tom would be of me. He watched finances carefully and was always on top of new and lower interest rates. The timing seemed appropriate since yesterday would have been our 30th wedding anniversary. It is like an anniversary present.

I also changed our financial advisory to my financial advisor. My new advisor gives me confidence that I have made the right decision and I feel that he communicates well while showing a genuine interest in my affairs. The office is also closer to home. I feel confident that it is time for growth in this area.

June 2009

Rachel and Bart came back to the Midwest for a visit. They are working on their house in Menomonie. Rachel asked if I could come and supervise the plumbing of the new sink. Bart did the work, and I offered the expertise, as it were. It was nice spending time with him.

A picnic was held at my house on the weekend so everyone could visit with Rachel and Bart, eliminating their need to run around to see everyone. The picnic was great fun. I realized how much I missed Rachel. All my children have always been a big part of my life and I do miss having them around.

June 25, 2009

Actress Farah Fawcett died today. Like many people, I was following her story, hoping for the best for her. Her cancer touched close to home for me. We both had anal cancer. At one time anal cancer was rarer than it is now. The scariest thing about anal cancer is that is tends to metastasize to the liver.

A young woman from Minneapolis, named Heidi, had anal cancer eight months before my diagnosis. After a year, she was told she was cancer free, much like Farah Fawcett had been told. Yet, a year later, they discovered that the cancer had metastasized to her liver and sadly, she too, died.

When medical professionals stress early detection they are so right. I found mine early thus allowing me the chance to be cured of my cancer and continue with my life.

July 2009

Larry has applied for Social Security Disability. With his combined spinal degeneration and diabetes, I think he may get it. They continue to have major difficulties in their lives, which continue to affect mine. I never expected them to live with me for so long. When the time is right for them, they will get a place of their own.

I am anxious to make life discoveries about myself once they do move. With them being such an integral part of my everyday life, I have not been able to do this.

August 2009

My daughter Val came for a visit from Oregon. Once again, we had a picnic so everyone could see Val and visit with her. It was a good visit. Valerie was here for her birthday, which was the first one I celebrated with her in three years.

Solution for Bladder Infections
September 2009

A few months ago, I did some research on bladder infections. The original use of cranberry juice is to prevent bacteria from attaching to the bladder wall and causing an infection. As I said, I had little luck with the cranberry juice.

I did; however, discover a supplement called D-Mannose with a cranberry extract. It serves the same function as cranberry juice. D-mannose is a simple sugar found naturally in birch and beech trees. D-Mannose removes the bad bacteria from your body by attaching to it and voiding the bad bacteria out through urination.

Unlike the cranberry juice, D-Mannose has been extremely effective for me. I have also combined the use of oil of oregano (strengthens the immune system) and Acidophilus.

Acidophilus has many health benefits such as protection against harmful bacteria, parasites, and other organisms. The hydrogen released by acidophilus creates a toxic environment for unhealthy creatures in our body and drives them out. It is helps with digestion by producing several chemicals, which aid digestion. In addition to digestive assistance, acidophilus is believed to help boost the immune system as a whole. It is also thought to provide some relief from intestinal problems, such as diarrhea.

My use of antibiotic for frequent bladder infections still had me concerned since antibiotics used to fight infections reduce the number of healthy flora (probiotic) in your system. Acidophilus can help replace these destroyed flora.

Instead of having a bladder infection every month I have not had one in three months since I started this supplement regiment.

I have also noticed that instead of getting up four or five times during the night to go to the bathroom, I get up only two or three times. The urgency pains have also gotten better, but I still have frequency and poor control during the day. I do not get as many loose and frequent loose stools as I once had. I have also increased my water intake each day. This helps to get rid of any urine that may be developing bacteria and resulting in a bladder infection.

I am completely used to wearing protective undergarments. I still do not like them, but they offer me freedom to be active away from home.

October 2009

I had my fourth Zometa IV treatment this month. I feel as though it is helping. I can tolerate my daily pain more easily making even the smallest improvement a Hg improvement. I will not have another bone density test until next year. I went to physical therapy in hopes it would improve my lower endurance and strength. I am afraid it will not be helpful. The exercise does not improve the pain or strength, so I am convinced the pain is from the bone and only time will improve that. I still exercise within my limits and feel some added strength in my legs, but not in my hips.

If it does not improve, I am fine with that. I have learned to do things differently, so I do not hurt myself or cause any undue pain. I walk with a cane, which prevents my hips and legs from tiring as quickly. I feel uncomfortable from time to time using it, but this too is an acceptance issue.

November 2009

I continue to make big strides in my journey toward a fulfilling and rewarding life. I miss Tom often, but the tears for his loss are far apart. When I was told that the pain from grief would lessen as time went by, I did not believe it could be possible. It is true. Even though I still miss Tom, the pain has lessened, and I can see continuing with my life without Tom. I enjoy pictures of him and conversations with others about his life.

After reading my journals I realized how vulnerable to other's whims I had become. The sorrow, depression and sadness were roadblocks to my recovery. Many of the words in my journal woke me up to the realization that I needed to cast off all of these roadblocks to my free my growth.

I survived vast turmoil over the past five years, and I learned many things about myself as well. I am a survivor, not only from cancer and loss, but also from physical limitations.

Shortly after Tom died, I truly believed I could not go on. I faced so many challenges in association with that nasty little word, cancer. It took my husband and some of my physical abilities.

After Tom died, someone asked me if I would have gone through cancer treatment knowing what I know now. Since I was so full of sorrow from Tom's loss, I said no. At that time, I felt my life was over because of all the ramifications of my journey through cancer.

I have changed my mind. I would have gone through it because I realize my role during Tom's treatments was so important. If I had died before him, he would have had to endure everything without me and died without my support. This was one purpose in my life.

If I had not survived, I would not have been able to give all the help and support I provided my parents over the past four years. I would have missed my daughter's wedding and I would not have been able to provide a home for Sandy and Larry in their time of need.

I can honestly say at this point in my life I do not know my purpose from day to day and that is fine. My purpose in life will find me because I am open to its appearance. When it enters my life, I will grab onto it and do the best with it that I can. I am alive and life will have a greater meaning for me than it ever has. I once heard that the purpose of life is to make a difference, even if it is only one life at a time. I have started with one life, my own.

Learning to date

What I have also discovered is that I do not like being alone as much as I am and have developed a fear of loneness or isolation.

I can only blame myself for this situation. Dating has taken on a new perspective for me. First, I haven't dating for over thirty years. I am a little rusty. Secondly, internet dating scares the heck out of me.

Since I have chosen isolation for much of the past few years, I am not surprised that I have not found a new relationship. For the first few years after Tom died, I felt as though I would be cheating on him if I dated. As I realized that it was not true or realistic to think this way, I knew that Tom would understand and want me to be happy in my life. I had to give myself permission to find personal happiness.

After getting that settled, I became fearful that I was not desirable enough for someone to what a relationship with me. I have some physical problems such as not being able to walk very far without pain and fatigue in my hips and legs. I am fearful of my lack of bladder and bowel control and fear that if the time was right, that physical intimacy would be painful.

As we age, many of us lose our perfectly healthy bodies. So, I concluded that I don't have to be perfect physically. If my perspective date cannot accept me as I am, he is not for me. I too must deal with the fact that maybe the right person for me will have some physical limitations as well. It can be dealt with if it is the right person.

My daughter Rachel and I discussed how I respond when I see someone who has possibilities. I told her that if they don't approach me, I don't respond at all. She simply said, "Mom, you need to remember how to flirt." She is right. Men do not have to make the first move. I remember flirting. Tom and I still did it even with our many years of marriage.

I concluded that I am now confident enough to flirt. Even though I am not yet dating, I am no longer in fear of being alone. I control it and I can make it happen. I can enjoy time with family and friends.

Wednesday, November 25, 2009

While visiting with a friend of mine at her office a man came in. I thought he looked familiar. After taking care of his business, he turned to me and asked if I was Tom's wife. I said yes and realized I now recognized him. We had a brief conversation about both Tom and my cancers. It was my cancer that he had further questions he wanted to ask.

His doctor had told him he had a fissure not to worry about it. His doctor recommended a high roughage diet and not to worry about it. (I heard those words before.) After hearing my story, the man decided that he was not going to take any chances and said he was going to have his doctor follow up on the fissure and have it repaired.

Whether he would have developed cancer in his colon if this injury were not repaired, I cannot say, but I feel strongly that it is not worth the chance. After I thought about the conversation, I realized that this too, might have been a purpose in my life resulting from my own cancer survival.

Life is worth Living
Sunday, December 27, 2009

The past five years have been a whirlwind of life-threatening disease, doctors, treatments and my husband's death. There were many times when I did not want to go on with my life. Many months of sorrow, depression and grief influenced me toward suicide, but the healing process has lessened those thoughts.

I cherish the wonderful memories of my life with Tom, and I find courage in doing this. I framed the last Valentine's card Tom gave to me and it sits near my computer along the polished red stone with the word LOVE carved upon it, that Tom gave me the same day. When I glance upon them, they make me smile as I remember how loved I had been by Tom.

I made many discoveries about myself, and my ability to survive. Within these discoveries, I learned that life is not easy, but life is worth living. It is worth fighting for no matter how challenging that fight may become.

Today I am free to live and free to celebrate that I am a cancer survivor.

Not all who get cancer survive. Not all who get cancer die. All who get cancer are truly unique people who must face a challenge of endurance, faith, hope and trust. My husband's struggle to live inspires me every day.

Today is December 27, 2009. Five years ago, today I became cancer free. Today, I am a true survivor.

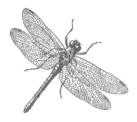

CHAPTER 18 – LIFE AFTER IT ALL

2010 – 2021

I used a half a box of tissue as I reviewed this manuscript. It was tough, but the tears released some of the lingering sorrow from over the past eleven years.

Time has a way of passing by without being truly noticed. Looking back, I am aware that I am not the same person I was when I first received my cancer diagnosis. I have changed physically, emotional, and spiritually.

Some of those changes are positive ones and some changes are challenging.

This final chapter is to share my survival from cancer and that of a widow.

Sandy and Larry found a place to call their home. I missed them for a while, but soon accepted living alone.

Dating

I never dated after Tom died. He was the love of my life, and I never felt the need to have another person in my life. I am not lonely even though I am alone. I may have days of feeling lonely, but that may be because I live alone. I value myself as a person and find many things to fill the time with activities.

I have gotten used to my singular routines and have been enjoying the freedom of having only myself to decide on the direction of my life. I am content with being by myself, which is not the same as being lonely.

I have come a long way along my path to recovery. Many

of the health problems I developed from cancer treatment are still a part of my life, but I have learned to accept them and deal with them in a positive way.

Some of the solutions I have discovered may be beneficial for others.

Dealing with Permanent Side Effects
Bladder and pelvic floor muscle damage - results and solutions

Radiation Therapy caused permanent damage to my pelvic floor muscles. I changed Urologists, which was for the better. I underwent several bladder tests to determine the capacity of my bladder, how much urine I released when I went pee, and my ability to hold my urgency.

Cystitis – UTI

I still have bladder incontinence due to the thickening of my bladder from both radiation and chemotherapy. Radiation therapy resulted in cystitis which is inflammation of the bladder wall. My cystitis is ongoing. I continue to use protective undergarments and have gotten used to the idea.

Due to pelvic floor muscle damage from radiation, my bladder only empties part of the urine. The remaining urine acts like a Petrie dish and grows e-coli. Since I cannot fully empty my bladder, I take a daily dose of antibiotic of which I have done for the past 16 years. To compensate for the loss of healthy flora in my intestines, I take large doses of multiple strains of both probiotic (acidophilus) and prebiotics. The combination is working, and I no longer have repeated UTI's.

Due to back surgery, I am unable to Cather myself and have no desire to let anyone else do it for me, as it would have to be daily. For now, the antibiotic is working quite well.

Radiation caused Peripheral artery disease

The front and back pelvic radiation damaged the arteries in both legs. This damage compromised the blood flow to both legs. The radiation damage is called Peripheral Artery disease of

PAD.

April 2011
First leg Artery emergency surgery

I had been experiencing strange sensations to my left leg. It would go numb to the touch, be extremely painful and become very cold. I had no idea what was happening but discovered that a heating blanket wrapped around my leg eased the pain. I treated it this way until one morning, it no longer helped.

When I woke that morning, my left was in such intense pain I could hear myself screaming. My sister Sandy and her husband took me to emergency, and I was then transported to a St Paul hospital for emergency surgery. The artery in my leg had collapsed.

Two five-inch stents were placed in my leg. I was put on a blood thinner, and things seemed much better.

2018 Second leg Artery surgery

Since I knew what to look for, I was aware when my right leg began to have the same systems as the left leg. I contacted my vascular surgeon. I was scheduled for a test on my legs.

The test consisted of using an ultrasound called a doppler to test the blood flow in the leg. I walked a tread mill and then the doppler and blood pressure cuffs were used.

The test indicated I had reduced blood flow when stationary, but almost no blood flow when active. My artery was collapsing.

Within two days I had my second stent surgery placing two five-inch stents in my right leg. I remain on a blood thinner, but the past few years it is the form of a daily dose of low dose aspirin.

Vascular Endothelial Cell Damage

The vascular endothelial cells form the inner lining of major blood cells. This helps form a smooth surface allowing blood to flow smoothly though the arteries. Radiation caused

damage to these cells, so the surfaces are no longer smooth causing calcified plaque to form in the arteries in my legs. This has
led to atherosclerosis.

Atherosclerosis

Atherosclerosis is the buildup of fats, cholesterol, and
other substances on the artery wall. This causing narrowing of
the arteries and reduced blood flow. My previous leg stent artery
placements were due to collapsed arteries (PAD) also caused by
radiation therapy.

Third Artery Surgery
April 2022

I have been having problems with my legs these past few
months. I had a doppler pressure test which led to a CT angiog-
raphy of my arms and legs. Contrast was used. Since my creatine
was slightly high the contrast was reduced to 75% of usual.

The result is that I am going to have surgery again to place
another stent in my left leg. My right leg blocked artery is in my
groin so stent cannot be used. They will use a patch and a tube
so they can move with my body. This procedure is called femoral
endarterectomy.

I hope the surgery and recovery go well.

This will be a lifelong challenge for me and I am looking
for alternative solutions to help heal my arteries.

Radiation Kidney Damage

Radiation therapy caused damaged to my kidneys. I had
expressed the pain I felt on both sides of my body, but it seemed
it was just thought to be pain from the cancer treatment.

It wasn't until I started IV treatment for bone damage
from radiation, that it was discovered that my kidneys were not
functioning in a healthy manner.

My creatine was higher than normal.

Nephrologist 2012

A nephrologist specializes in kidney disease.

After seeing the nephrologist, my IV treatment for osteoporosis was discontinued. The drug I was on was causing further damage to my radiation damaged kidneys.

Currently, I am late stage 3 kidney disease. I am on a renal diet which is a strict diet to be on. Once again, the strength within you will come forward and help with yet another challenge. I remained hopeful that the kidney disease will not progress.

Be sure to discuss with your doctor any steps you can take to help protect other parts of your body while undergoing radiation therapy.

Both chemotherapy and radiation therapy can cause permanent side effects. When you discuss the possible side effects from treatment be sure to ask about any permanent side effects that might occur. Be sure to ask what steps you can take to lessen any permanent side effects. It could be as simple as more water intake, certain supplements, or other medications.

Any steps to help protect your body, whether it is organs or bones, is worth pursuing.

Osteoporosis 2016

Radiation therapy caused damage to the bones in my lower back and pelvis bones. I was on an oral medication for it, but when I didn't show improvement after two years, I went to an IV medication. I had this medication once every six months. Before each IV treatment my creatine was checked to see if my kidneys could handle the treatment. The nurse noticed that my kidney function decreased with each treatment.

I went to the Nephrologist who ultimately stopped the IV treatment.

In 2016 I required lower back surgery to repair deteriorated bones. The surgery included four screws in my spine and a bone fusion to the lower spine. I was told they would use a cadaver bone since the bone they would have used would have come from my pelvis. Osteoporosis in my pelvis made that impossible.

After surgery, I was told that they were able to use bone from my pelvis since they did not see any osteoporosis present. I very pleasantly surprise. The back surgery vastly improved the quality of my life.

I have come to terms with permanent side effects from cancer treatment. I was asked if, I knew that I would have these lifelong problems before cancer treatment would I have done it?

Even though radiation therapy has caused damage to many systems and parts of my body, I would have considered medication and supplements that could have added more protection to the damage areas.

Both radiation and chemotherapy have given me the additional years that I am living, and I am grateful for that. Dealing with some of the latent side effects is a lifelong process and I do the best I can with each day.

So, the answer is yes, yes, yes! I have experience so many wonderful things over the past 17 years because I did survive. Even though I continued to live without Tom, I would not have wanted to miss out on those wonderful memories. I can "live" with my medical conditions because the key world is – live.

Emotional Recovery as widow and cancer survivor

When Tom first died, I thought the pain and grief I felt would never lessen. It does take time and each person needs to grieve in their own way and at their own pace. I still grieve for Tom, but the pain is no longer as devastating as it had been.

I can remember good times we had and smile. I can look at pictures and smile. I will always miss him. I still try to live for both of us, in his memory.

There are times when I really wish I could share experiences with him such as our children's wedding and the birth of our grandsons.

The birth of my first grandson, Remy was my life saver. His birth filled the emptiness I felt for Tom with pure happiness and purpose. When Ivan was born, I was twice blessed.

RITA K MILLER KASINSKAS

All thoughts of suicide disappeared the day Remy was born and have never returned. I think the man in my life that Tom was sending to me was my grandsons. They have made my life more complete than it has in a long time.

Even though it took me a while, I can now celebrate that I am a cancer survivor. I no longer feel guilty that I lived, and Tom died.

I am thankful that I lived so I could experience the many joys I have over the past years.

I am thankful that I could be present to be helpful to my aging parents and be instrumental to support them in their illness. I am grateful I was present to help them both die with dignity when their time came.

My father died in September 2011 from cancer. It then became my sister, Sandy, and me to care for our mother. This included daily trips to dialysis, cooking, cleaning, and caring for her. It was demanding, but I am grateful I survived my cancer so I could help care for her. She died in September 2016 from a heart attack.

My two nieces both survived their thyroid cancer. My brother-in-law Al, did find sobriety the last few years of his life, but sadly dies of COPD in 2019.

I still fill some of my time helping others. I do this because I want to, not out of obligation. I have learned to say no and choose whether to help or not. Keeping myself happy and positive allows me to do the same for others.

This way, I know I am living my life for me and not for others.

It is very GOOD to be alive.

Financial Recovery
Employment and Financial

Even though I was on Social Security Disability I wanted to return to some type of employment. I obtained a part time position as a receptionist. That went on for almost two. The employment ended after my back surgery as it seemed like too much for me to return at that time.

I am now on regular Social Security and have no interest in becoming employed again. Caring for my grandchild helped to satisfy my productivity need and it is a lot more fun!

I have adjusted my spending so I can afford to live on Social Security. I have some small investments that serve as an emergency parachute for sudden and unexpected home repairs or used car purchase.

The ten-year plan I put into place elven years ago, resulted in the satisfaction of my home mortgage in December 2021. A very great accomplishment of which I know Tom smiled about.

I now have a wonderful peace of mind that I can make it from month to month and live comfortably. Not fancy, but comfortable.

Life Is Worth Living

Throughout our lives we will be facing many difficult situations that we may feel we can never survive. I have been there may times throughout the past 17 years.

We are very resilient people and are capable of more than we may imagine.

Remember, there is a strength within you that you may not realize you have. Many people find this strength through their faith, from family and friends and others find this strength by believing in themselves, that they can survive.

I hope by sharing my seventeen-year journey with you, that you find the strength within yourself and know that you can overcome so many challenges and struggles within your life. It is amazing, how the strength and belief within yourself will help you to become a survivor of anything.

ABOUT THE AUTHOR

Rita K. Kasinskas

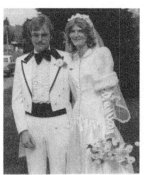 Rita K. Miller married Thomas J. Kasinskas on May 19, 1979. The had three children and lived in rural Wisconsin.

Rita is an entrepreneur, journalist, columnist, artist, and author. She still lives in rural Wisconsin and enjoys nature and American Indian history and culture. The highlights of her life are her children and her two grandsons of whom she sees often.

BOOKS BY THIS AUTHOR

The White Buffalo's Feather - Fiction Novel

When dreams which are part of everyday life, mystically become reality, adventures begin.

Deseray's adventures begin, first with a reoccuring dream riding upon the back of a great white buffalo and continue upon meeting a young American Indian man, Reg, a white buffalo and receiving a mystical eagle's feather. This sparked her desire to learn and understand about the original native people of America.

She goes on an archaeological dig in Montana with her uncle John. The anonymous sponsor of the dig adds to the intrigue of her adventure. While on the dig, the mystical powers of the buffalo's eagle feather transports her to times past when the prairies were home to the American Indian.

Fulfilling her desire to learn about their way of life, she discovers that the days were filled with hard work, struggles for survival and traditional activities of their daily life. She also learns many of their customs, family values and sacred rituals.

Unexpectantly, she also discovers love. The young American Indian man she had met in her own time, Tall Trees, who became her guide in the past.

As time passed, she learned much about these wonderful people and learned to love them. Often, she wondered if she would ever return to her own time. Part of her wanted to remain in the past forever, and another part of her wanted to go back to her own time and her home.

UNTITLED

Made in the USA
Middletown, DE
17 April 2022